The Psychiatrist's Guide to Capitation and Risk-Based Contracting

The Psychiatrist's Guide to Capitation and Risk-Based Contracting

American Psychiatric Association

Office of Economic Affairs and Practice Management

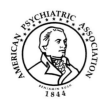

Other monographs on managed care available from the APA Office of Economic Affairs and Practice Management:

The Psychiatrist's Managed Care Primer (Order #2450)
The Psychiatrist's Guide to Practice Management (Order #2451)
The Psychiatrist's Guide to Managed Care Contracting (Order #2454)
The Psychiatrist's Guide to Capitation and Risk-Based Contracting (Order #2453)
Public Mental Health: A Changing System in an Era of Managed Care (Order #2452)
American Psychiatric Association Capitation Handbook (Order #2277)

To order, please contact:

American Psychiatric Press, Inc.
1400 K Street, N.W.
Washington, DC 20005
www.appi.org
1-800-368-5777
fax: 202-789-2648
e-mail: order@appi.org

Copyright © 1997
American Psychiatric Association
ALL RIGHTS RESERVED
Manufactured in the United States of America on acid-free paper
First Edition
00 99 98 97
4 3 2 1

American Psychiatric Association
1400 K Street, N.W.
Washington, DC 20005

Library of Congress Cataloging-in-Publication Data
The psychiatrist's guide to capitation and risk-based contracting / by American Psychiatric Association Office of Economic Affairs and Practice Management.
      p.   cm.
    Includes bibliographical references.
    ISBN 0-89042-453-5 (alk. paper)
    1. Psychiatry—Practice—United States.   2. Capitation fees (Medical care).   3. Insurance, Mental health—United States.   4. Risk (Insurance).   I. American Psychiatric Association. Office of Economic Affairs and Practice Management.
    [DNLM: 1. Psychiatry—organization & administration.
2. Capitation Fee—organization & administration.   3. Managed Care Programs—organization & administration.   4. Professional Practice—organization & administration.   WM 21 P9736 1997]
RC465.6.P778   1997
616.89'0068—dc21
DNLM/DLC
for Library of Congress
                                                                97-12762
                                                                CIP

British Library Cataloguing in Publication Data
A CIP record is available from the British Library.

Table of Contents

I	Introduction	1

II	Capitation Models Currently Employed in Mental Health	3
	A Capitation and the Changing Practice Environment	3
	B Full Risk and Partial Risk Capitation	7
	C Limiting Financial Risk	9

III	Understanding Capitation Rate Development	13
	A Population Characteristics	13
	B Benefit Plan Characteristics	15
	C Scope of Covered Services	16
	D Utilization Factors	16
	E Costs of Services	17
	F Capitation Rate Structure	17
	1 Budgetary Method	17
	2 Fee-for-Service Method	18
	3 Basic Components of a Capitation Rate	18

G	Cost of Clinical Services	19
H	Estimating the Number of Services	19
I	Estimating the Cost per Unit of Service	21
J	Estimating Overhead Costs	23
K	Profit and Capital Allowances	25
L	Sample Capitation Rate Calculation	25
	1 *Step One: Determine the Benefit Plan and Member Group*	25
	2 *Step Two: Determine the Utilization Rates for the Group*	26
	3 *Step Three: Determine the Costs of Services*	26
	4 *Step Four: Determine the Costs of Overhead Requirements*	29
	5 *Step Five: Determine the Profit Expectation*	31
	6 *Step Six: Test for Reasonableness*	31

IV Evaluating and Negotiating a Capitation Contract

			35
A	Assessment of the Proposed Capitation Rate		35
B	Operational Terms of the Contract		36
	1	*Payment Provisions*	36
	2	*Duties of the Psychiatric Practice*	38
	3	*Duties of the MCO*	39
	4	*General Provisions*	40
C	Understanding Benefit Exclusions		41
D	Dispute Resolution and/or Procedures for "Gray Area" Services		42
E	Checklist for Evaluating Capitated Agreements		43
	1	*Introductory Contract Provisions*	43
	2	*Compensation*	44
	3	*Psychiatrist Duties*	45
	4	*MCO Duties*	48
	5	*Other Considerations*	49
	6	*Boilerplate Language*	50

V	**Organizational and Administrative Issues in Managing a Capitated Contract**	53
	A Clinical Management Issues	53
	B Network Development and Maintenance	54
	1 *Composition and Geographic Distribution*	54
	2 *Credentialing*	55
	3 *Training and Communication*	55
	C Administrative Processes	56
	1 *Claims Processing*	57
	2 *Appeals Process*	57
	3 *Quality Improvement*	58
	D Management Information Systems	59
	1 *General MIS Requirements*	60
	E Financial Monitoring	67
	1 *Capitation Reconciliation*	67
	2 *Claims Payment*	67
	3 *Claims Expense and IBNR Calculation*	68
	4 *Financial Reporting*	68
VI	**Legal and Regulatory Issues for Capitated Psychiatrists**	71
VII	**The Dilemma of Quality in Capitated Systems**	75
	A The Conflict of Incentives	75
	B Satisfaction and Outcomes Measures	76
VIII	**Conclusion**	79
IX	**Appendix 1 Determination of Claim Liability: Medical vs. Psychiatrist Claims**	81

| x | Appendix 2 | Instructions for Using the Capitation Worksheet to Estimate a Capitation Rate | 87 |

| XI | APA Resources and Services for Psychiatrists Working in Managed Care | 93 |

| XII | Capitation and Risk-Based Contracting Bibliography | 95 |

| XIII | Capitation and Risk-Based Contracting Glossary | 97 |

Introduction

In today's competitive economic environment, many psychiatric practitioners are electing to enter capitation agreements with managed care organizations or other payers. In these agreements, psychiatrists share some or assume all of the financial risk related to the care they are contracted to provide to a given population. In this monograph on capitation and its companion disk, we provide some of the tools essential to developing a successful capitated program, including a summary of the primary financial, administrative, and clinical issues involved in such a contract. We hope that this monograph will facilitate the decisions made by psychiatrists in achieving a successful capitation contract.

The APA would like to express its appreciation to Open Minds for its assistance preparing this document, to Robert T.M. Phillips, M.D., Ph.D., for making this project a reality, and to the following consultant advisors for lending their expertise:

> Jeremy Lazarus, M.D.
> David Pruitt, M.D.
> Chester Schmidt, M.D.
> Nancy Wheeler, J.D.

I would also like to thank the staff of the Office of Economic Affairs and Practice Management for their countless hours coordinating the project, conducting research, and editing and drafting text to make these products as useful as possible:

> Mary Graham, Director
> Sajini Thomas, Health Economist

Katherine Moore, Health Economist
Carolyn Heier, Industry Analyst
Jesse Gately, Research Assistant
Donna Hagler, Administrative Assistant

I am pleased to add this monograph to the APA's array of products designed to be valuable resources in coping with capitated contracts.

Melvin Sabshin, M.D.

Melvin Sabshin, M.D.
Medical Director

Capitation Models Currently Employed in Mental Health

A. Capitation and the Changing Practice Environment

The continued expansion of managed care has brought with it fundamental changes in the way psychiatrists are paid for services. In the past, psychiatrists were paid on a fee-for-service basis for a specific type and amount of service. Now, managed care practices are transferring increasing financial risk to the psychiatrist and psychiatric practice. The most risk-intensive form of payment is "capitation," whereby a psychiatrist or psychiatric practice receives a flat payment per beneficiary or per patient to provide all mental health services needed by members of a group within their defined benefit plan. Acceptance of a capitation contract places the practitioner at risk for provision, either through direct delivery or through contract delivery, of all services needed by the members of the insured group, no matter how much and no matter what the cost.

Capitation Payment Illustration

- Number of Covered Members: **25,000**
- Psychiatry Capitation Rate per Member per Month: **$3.75**
- Capitation Payment per Month: **$93,750**

Capitation is often called a "population-based" payment method because the psychiatrist or psychiatric group is paid an amount per member for all members in a covered group. (Throughout this monograph, the examples will refer to a psychiatric group practice considering capitation.) An example of a capitation payment is illustrated above.

3

II

In this example, a psychiatrist or psychiatric group would receive $93,750 each month to provide all of the psychiatric services used by the 25,000 members during that month. (This example assumes that the psychiatric group is responsible for all mental health services defined in the benefit plan.)

As a method of financing, capitation has an extensive history beginning perhaps with the first prepaid healthcare arrangement provided by the Sisters of Charity in Galveston, Texas, in the early 1900s. For $1 per month, the hospital would provide any necessary medical care to the families of seamen operating out of the port of Galveston. Zieman cites the first employee carve-out occurring in 1910 at the Western Clinic in Tacoma, Washington.[1] For $0.50 per member per month, the Western Clinic provided all necessary medical care to the employees of a local lumber mill. The emergence of the "company hospital" and the "company doctor" in industries such as railroads and mining in the early part of the century were also nascent models of capitation. One major national managed care company, the Kaiser Permanente Health Plan, has its roots in this movement.

The growth of managed care in mental health services is illustrated in Figure 1. Overall, the best market share estimates show a growth in the number of insured citizens in managed mental health care programs of at least 25% since 1993.[2]

In data published by the InterStudy Group, an organization devoted to the study of managed care and health maintenance organizations (HMOs), approximately 57% of enrolled members in 1995 were in HMOs that reimbursed psychiatrists under capitated models.

With these historical roots, the growth of managed care to modern day levels has brought new methods of financing to the forefront for many psychiatrists, either directly through new capitation agreements or indirectly through membership in capitated managed care networks.

---

[1] Zieman, G. "Nearly a Century of Capitation: How and Why," *The Complete Capitation Handbook,* 1995, page 1.
[2] *Managed Behavioral Health Market Share in the United States,* 1996–1997.

||

Table 1 describes key payment types besides capitation in order of increasing financial risk to the psychiatrist or psychiatric practice. The services of an actuary with familiarity in mental health capitation issues should be used to evaluate the appropriateness of a capitation rate and the eventual risk liability for the psychiatric practice.

Once the psychiatric practice accepts payment arrangements other than some fee-for-service variant, a fundamental change in thinking is required for success. This type of reimbursement mechanism requires that the psychiatric practice shift its perspective from the needs of the individual patient to the needs of the entire covered group of members. For example, these contracts usually specify a time period within which a member requesting services must be seen. The traditional method of dealing with excessive demand—the "waiting list"—is not an option under capitation. In the event of excessive demand, the psychiatric practice must make alternative arrangements for the patients' care, either through increasing its capacity or contracting with other psychiatrists for the services. Payment for these contracted services must come from the psychiatric practice's capitation, not from additional funds from the payer.

Managed Mental Health Care on the Increase

FIGURE 1

Number of U.S. Citizens in Managed Mental Health Programs, in Millions

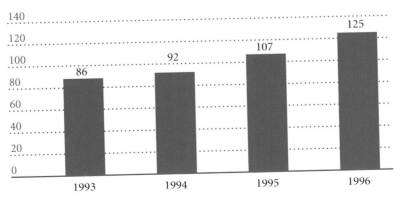

Source: Managed Behavioral Health Market Share in the United States, 1996–1997.

II

TABLE 1

Payment Methodology

Payment Methodology	Definition	Type of Risk to the Psychiatric Practice
Fee-for-Service (FFS)	The psychiatric practice is reimbursed usual and customary charges for services rendered.	This method has risk for the psychiatric practice only to the extent that the amount charged covers the direct costs, indirect costs, and profit goals per unit of service for the psychiatric practice. In addition, the psychiatric practice must be able to bill for sufficient services to meet overall practice costs and income needs.
Discounted Fee-for-Service	The psychiatric practice is reimbursed some percentage of usual and customary charges. In most cases, the discount given ranges from 10% to 20% of the usual charge.	The risk of this method is essentially the same as fee-for-service.
Fee Schedule	The psychiatric practice is reimbursed according to a set schedule of fees, usually by CPT code. These rates are usually set by the insurer, based on local, regional, or national cost and payment patterns. (An example is the Resource-Based Relative Value Scale.) These fees may or may not have any relation to the psychiatric practice's usual and customary charges, although they are almost always below them. This is the most common method employed by managed behavioral health care companies.	The risk of this method is essentially the same as fee-for-service.
Partial Capitation	Under this method, the psychiatric practice is paid a fixed fee per member per month for all members enrolled in a benefit plan. The payment is called a partial capitation in that it typically covers only a limited set of services, usually professional services. Other services, such as hospitalization or referral to other specialists, are not covered by the capitation.	Next to full capitation, this shifts the maximum amount of risk to the psychiatric practice in that the rate implies full responsibility for the delivery of a defined set of services to a group of covered members. If the psychiatric practice's capacity is insufficient to meet the need of presenting covered members, other arrangements must be made by the psychiatric practice to ensure that member needs are met.

II

The need for a change in thinking is best illustrated by comparing the traditional incentives of fee-for-service to the new incentives under capitation. Under fee-for-service, the amount of profit is driven by increasing the units of service delivered. This incentive of "the more you do, the more you make" is often cited as a major weakness of indemnity insurance, the traditional health care financing mechanism. Capitation shifts the profit-making incentives, with increasing units of service lowering the amount of profits.

The primary cause of this change is the relative constancy of the revenue. Because capitation is a fixed fee per member per month (PMPM), the total revenue changes only with fluctuations in membership. Therefore, the delivery of increasing units of services does not produce increasing revenue, only increasing costs and decreasing profits. The incentive to "deliver less to make more" is often cited as the principal drawback of capitation. Underserving patients is the criticism most often leveled at managed mental health care companies and HMOs in general.

The administration of a capitation contract and the delivery of quality services are not mutually exclusive. They do, however, demand new organizational and clinical capabilities.

B.   Full Risk and Partial Risk Capitation

Under the capitation method of payment, psychiatrists are paid a set amount PMPM for those patients who elect or are assigned to receive covered services through the psychiatric practice. Capitated payment for services comes either directly through a contract with an insurer or MCO or through "subcapitation" from a contractor organization responsible for providing mental health services for the health plan's members (also known as a "carve-out").

Under the first model, the MCO or primary payer contracts directly with the psychiatric practice for covered mental health services. When this type of capitation contracting is used for the entire mental health benefit, the capitation contract usually requires that the group practice have a network of clinicians and facilities under contract able to provide the full range of needed services.

The fixed capitated payment has no direct relationship to the actual amount of services provided to beneficiaries. Rather, the payment is a predetermined amount paid for each member of the plan that is intended to adequately compensate the psychiatric practice for all covered services provided to the members for that month. Because the payment is a fixed amount, the psychiatric practice is accepting risk for the potential overutilization of services by patients and for the cost of providing services for catastrophic individual cases. In the alternative, the psychiatric practice may also benefit from underutilization of services and the absence of catastrophic cases.

In some mental health carve-outs, the psychiatric practice is capitated only for its direct professional services. This payment method is often referred to as a partial capitation or a subcapitation. The payment is not intended to cover other services such as treatment provided by other professionals or inpatient hospitalization services.

The variability of "covered services" in a capitation contract demands careful review by the psychiatric practice before acceptance of such a contract. Failure to completely understand the nature of the services covered by the capitation can lead to financial disaster as the psychiatric practice discovers it is responsible for payment of services not directly delivered or controlled in the practice.

Once the "flow" of premium dollars is established, there are two methods for determining the actual capitation rate paid to the psychiatric practice. One method for establishing PMPM capitation rates is to pay the psychiatric practices per member a certain percentage of the monthly premium for all medical care. Although not widely used in determining mental health capitation rates, this method has additional risk in that the increasingly competitive health care market is demanding that MCOs either maintain their current premium rates or decrease them. Because monthly premium charges may not increase, and may decrease, this may not be the best way to determine psychiatrist capitation. In other words, a psychiatrist should not necessarily receive less money just because an MCO may decide not to increase its premium. Further, in accepting a certain percentage of the monthly premium as capitation, the psychiatric practice is accepting the actuarial determination and assumptions made by the MCO, without the input of the psychiatric practice's own actuarial analysis. In addition, the use of percentage of premium capitation payments may raise legal issues, since it may be prohibited under some state insurance laws.

The more common method for determining the PMPM capitation rate in mental health uses more direct analysis of the historical utilization of services by members coupled with an estimate of the cost to provide those services. Using this method, the psychiatric practice attempts to predict the number of patients requesting services, the numbers and types of services those members may need, and the unit costs of each service.

C.   Limiting Financial Risk

There are two primary ways a psychiatric practice can limit the risk in a capitation contract: (1) acquisition of stop-loss insurance; and (2) negotiation of a risk corridor in the contract. Stop-loss insurance is a form of reinsurance that provides protection for medical expenses above a certain limit, either on a per-case basis or in the aggregate on an annual basis. The term "stop-loss coverage" has traditionally been used in the medical services arena, providing loss protection to independent practice associations (IPAs), medical groups, and other physician arrangements. The synonym "reinsurance" has traditionally been used in the hospital services arena, providing this coverage for hospitals. Stop-loss insurance can be purchased from the psychiatrist's current insurer or the payer.

A risk corridor is a provision in the capitation contract in which the payer, in this example an HMO, agrees to share the risk with the psychiatrist within a specified range. For example, a risk corridor provision might call for the HMO and the psychiatric practice to share the costs of care if the cost per member per month (PMPM) exceeds some target. An example is stated below.

II

The capitation rate is established at $4 PMPM. The HMO has agreed to a risk corridor provision in which the HMO will share costs on a graduated basis with the psychiatric practice as shown in Table 2.

Using the example shown in Table 2, the costs for the downside risk to the psychiatric practice would be limited as shown in Table 3.

The downside to a risk corridor provision in a contract with the HMO is that in exchange for providing some downside risk coverage, the HMO will often want to share in any upside profits, usually on the same percentage basis.

Specific examples of how different forms of stop-loss function are provided in Table 4.

Stop-loss provisions have been incorporated into many capitated psychiatrist contracts as a mechanism to limit the psychiatric practice's

TABLE 2

Per Member per Month Costs—Percentages

Cost per Member per Month	HMO Risk-Sharing Portion	Psychiatrist Risk-Sharing Portion
$4	0%	100%
$4.25	20%	80%
$4.50	35%	65%
$4.75	50%	50%
$5 and higher	80%	20%

TABLE 3

Per Member per Month Costs—Dollars

Cost per Member per Month	HMO Risk-Sharing Portion	Psychiatrist Risk-Sharing Portion	Ultimate Capitation Cost to the Psychiatrist
$4	$0.000	$0.000	$4.000
$4.25	$0.050	$0.200	$4.200
$4.50	$0.175	$0.325	$4.325
$4.75	$0.375	$0.375	$4.375
$5 and higher	$0.60 (0.05+0.175+0.375) plus 80% of costs exceeding $5	$0.90 (0.20+0.325+0.375) plus 20% of costs exceeding $5	$4.900 plus 20% of costs exceeding $5

II

financial risk for individual catastrophic cases and treatment programs or procedures that greatly exceed the PMPM capitation payment.

Once a dollar limit is reached for services provided either to a particular patient or in the aggregate, the stop-loss coverage will then cover a certain percentage of costs above the dollar limit. Because MCOs may indirectly charge psychiatrists for the stop-loss protection, psychiatrists may wish to instead obtain separate stop-loss coverage through a reinsurance company.

The Individual Stop-Loss Program ("ISL") is designed to limit the psychiatric practice's risk for capitated services under capitated health plans per member per calendar year to a specified amount (the "Deductible"). In this example, the HMO shall reimburse the psychiatric practice at eighty percent (80%) of the fee-for-service rates in excess of the Deductible. Capitated services shall be valued at the fee-for-service rates for purposes of determining whether the ISL Deductible has been met. The HMO shall deduct two percent (2%) from the psychiatric practice's capitation payment each month for participation in the ISL program.

Stop-Loss Arrangements

TABLE 4

Stop-Loss Arrangement	Actual Costs	Maximum Risk to the Psychiatric Practice	Amount Paid by the Stop-Loss Arrangement
Per Case Basis ($50,000 stop-loss coverage)	$75,000 for one case	$50,000	$25,000
Aggregate Basis (Coverage in excess of 125% of premium for a premium of $3.00 pmpm for 20,000 lives)	$840,000 or $3.50 pmpm × 12 months (116% of premium)	$840,000 or $3.50 pmpm × 12 months (There is still $60,000 of liability remaining before hitting the stop-loss threshold of 125%)	$0.00
Aggregate Basis (Coverage in excess of 125% of premium for a premium of $3.00 pmpm for 20,000 lives)	$1,020,000 or $4.25 pmpm × 12 months (142% of premium)	$900,000 or $3.75 pmpm × 12 months (125% of premium)	$120,000 or $0.50 pmpm × 12 months (The 17% of premium over the 125% stop-loss limit)

II

TABLE 5

Sample Stop-Loss Arrangements

Item	Calculation
Psychiatrist's Capitation	$3.00 pmpm ($36 pmpy)
Deduction for Stop Loss	2% or $0.06 ($0.72 pmpy)
Net Capitation Rate	$2.94 ($35.28 pmpy)
Annual Revenue (20,000 members)	$705,600
Deductible Point	$39.60 pmpy (110% of capitation)
Actual Cost of Care	$850,000 or $42.50 pmpy
80% of the Amount in Excess of the Deductible	$2.32 pmpy (($42.50 - 39.60) \times .80$)
Amount Due Psychiatrist From Stop-Loss Claim	$46,400 ($2.32 \times 20,000$)
Loss to Psychiatrist Before Stop-Loss	$144,400 ($0.612 pmpm)
Loss After Stop-Loss Payment	$98,000 ($0.408 pmpm)

The psychiatric practice must submit ISL claims in accordance with the HMO's policies and procedures manual. Such claims must be submitted no later than ninety (90) days from the end of the calendar year in order to be credited to the ISL program. The HMO will pay all ISL claims within ninety (90) days of receipt of a properly submitted claim.

Services where payment is received from any third party, such as a workers' compensation carrier or other primary insurance, and member copayments are not considered costs for purposes of calculating the ISL Deductible.

An illustration of the above stop-loss provision is shown in Table 5.

Understanding Capitation Rate Development

This section will explain the basics of capitation rate development using two models: the budgetary model and the fee-for-service method. Before illustrating these methods, an examination of the factors affecting capitation rate development must be discussed.

In preparing an actuarial analysis of capitation rates, various factors that affect the determination of the rate of capitation for a psychiatric practice should be considered. These factors include the following:

- Characteristics of the covered population such as size, type of industry, and age and sex of the members;

- The type of benefit plan being offered, including copayment, deductible, and out-of-pocket requirements;

- The exact scope of services included in and excluded from the capitation rate;

- The projected number of members utilizing services and the type and number of services used; and

- The costs of services to be delivered.

A.   Population Characteristics

HMOs traditionally take the age and sex of members into account in determining rates by making tiered capitation rates, which vary based on both of these factors. These methods are not commonly used in

III

determining mental health capitation rates, however, because of the lack of industry-wide utilization benchmarks. As the industry collects more data from mental health capitation arrangements, this may become a more relevant factor.

Of greater relevance is the size of the population for which the psychiatric practice is accepting capitation. Generally, the larger the group size, the more predictable the utilization and thus the more predictable the risk. Capitation for a group of 100,000 members is easier to evaluate and manage than capitation for a group of 1,000. This results from the "law of large numbers" and the relative size of the standard deviation from the norm. Simply stated, the "law of large numbers" holds that the *actual* outcome of a statistical process converges toward the *expected* value as the number of observations increase.[3] Table 6 illustrates this point.

As demonstrated, the deviation from the expected cost, and thus the eventual financial risk, decreases as the number of covered lives increases.

For this reason, if the HMO has low membership enrollment in the service area in which the psychiatric practice will provide services, some psychiatrist contracts provide for a minimum number of members who must be enrolled in the HMO health plan in the service area before the psychiatric practice is paid on a PMPM capitated basis.

---

[3] Ryan, J.B. & Clay, S.B. "Understanding the Law of Large Numbers," Healthcare Financial Management, 1995, Volume 49, No. 10, page 22.

TABLE 6   **Expected Costs of Hospitalizations**

Per Member per Month	Number of Covered Lives			
	100	1,000	10,000	20,000
Expected Cost	$26.28	$26.28	$26.28	$26.28
Standard Deviation of Expected Cost	$34.67	$10.96	$3.47	$1.55

III

B. Benefit Plan Characteristics

The type of benefit plan being considered has a direct effect on the capitation rate based on the following factors:

Traditional HMO

- Characteristics—Closed network of psychiatrists; all services must be pre-authorized; fixed dollar copayments; service limits (i.e., 20 visits, 30 days); and no out-of-network coverage.

- Effect on capitation rate—The capitation rate is easier to calculate because of the lack of benefits for services not pre-authorized and not delivered by a network psychiatrist. Also, the value of copayments are fixed regardless of the cost of service.

Preferred Provider Organization (PPO) and Point of Service (POS) Plans

- Characteristics—In- and out-of-network psychiatrists; some coverage extended for non-authorized services; and percentage copayments.

- Effect on capitation rate—Rate is more difficult to calculate due to the presence of coverage for non-authorized services and out-of-network psychiatrists. Copayment value is dependent upon the cost of service.

Also, the specific features of the benefit plan can affect the capitation rate as follows:

Copayment level The higher the copayment level, the lower the capitation rate as the copayment is subtracted from the unit cost of the service.

Deductible level The higher the deductible level, the lower the capitation rate as the deductible is subtracted from the cost of the service or the cost of the episode of care.

Covered services The broader the range of covered services, the higher the capitation level.

In addition, an increase in the copayment and deductible levels will tend to decrease utilization.

C.   Scope of Covered Services

It is important to specifically define in detail the nature and scope of the benefit plan before entering into a capitation arrangement. Failure to understand the intricacies of benefit plan coverage can lead to negative financial results if the psychiatric practice must provide more services than anticipated in the capitation rate. The following example questions illustrate the importance of this point:

- Is chemical dependency treatment covered? If so, who is responsible for the costs of medical detoxification?

- What is the limit on the benefits? For example, is the outpatient benefit limited to a certain number of visits or a certain aggregate dollar cost?

- Are there any exclusions to coverage such as treatment for AIDS dementia, court-ordered treatment, testing for learning disabilities, etc.?

- Who is responsible for psychiatric consultations for a patient on a medical floor hospitalized for a physical medical condition?

In Chapter IV, Evaluating and Negotiating a Capitated Contract, the full range of these issues will be discussed.

D.   Utilization Factors

Obviously, the estimates of how many members are going to use what and how many services are of prime importance in determining a capitation rate. In most cases, the psychiatric practice will want to obtain the prior utilization history of the covered group to assist in making these projections. In some cases, however, the utilization history will not be available, as in the case of a newly covered group

III

or a new HMO, or it will not be directly applicable, as in the case of a group moving from a free-choice indemnity plan to a tightly managed HMO plan. If possible, it is most desirable to obtain the raw claims data experience for the group so that the psychiatric practice and/ or the consulting actuary can analyze the exact nature of the historical utilization. Although more time consuming, analysis of the actual claims data yields a greater range of information than that provided on standard utilization reports.

E.   Costs of Services

As with utilization history, the detailed knowledge of the cost of services to be provided is vital to the development of an accurate capitation rate. Here, history of costs is not directly applicable, as the psychiatric practice must calculate the value of the services it plans to deliver under the capitation arrangement. If a network of psychiatrists other than the psychiatric practice is required, the contract rates to be paid under the contract must be known.

F.   Capitation Rate Structure

Given these variables, a capitation rate can be calculated using either a budgetary method or a fee-for-service method.

F.1.   Budgetary Method

The budgetary method projects the costs of services and translates this cost into full-time-equivalent (FTE) psychiatrists required "per 1,000" covered lives. These staffing requirements should be adjusted for each of the various subspecialties required to meet the needs of patients, and they should include the necessary overhead personnel and administrative costs required to support the activities of psychiatrists.[4]

---

[4] Sutton, H.L. & Sorbo, A.J. Actuarial Issues in the Fee-for-Service/Prepaid Medical Group, Center for Research in Ambulatory Health Care Administration, Englewood, CO, 1993, page 29.

III

A simple example of this method for a 20,000 member group is presented in Table 7.

This calculation can be expanded to include projected utilization rates by psychiatric subspecialty and to account for utilization of services by non-psychiatrists in cases where the psychiatric practice uses a network of psychiatrists. In addition, the rate should be expanded to include hospital visits, overhead costs, and an allowance for profit and capital costs. These costs can be allocated to the cost of an FTE or converted to per 1,000 units to add to the PMPM rate.

F.2. Fee-for-Service Method

The more common method of determining the capitation rate is the fee-for-service method, which projects the cost of services delivered based on the contracted or calculated costs per unit of service. The projected utilization of different types of services is combined with the projected costs per unit of service to yield a total cost translated into a PMPM rate. This method will be used to illustrate the development of a hypothetical capitation rate further in this section.

F.3. Basic Components of a Capitation Rate

In general, a capitation rate will have the following basic components:

- The estimated cost of direct clinical services, expressed as a PMPM number.

TABLE 7   **Capitation Calculation**

Item	Calculation	Result
Assumed Utilization Rate for Outpatient Psychiatry	0.1 psychiatrist visits per year (10% penetration rate)	
Assumed Productivity Rate	3,000 office visits per psychiatrist per year	
Psychiatrist FTE Need	$3,000 \div 0.1$	1 FTE per 30,000 members or 0.033 FTEs per 1,000 members
Cost of Psychiatry FTE	$175,000	
Cost per Member per Month	$(0.033 \times 175,000) \div (1,000 \times 12)$	$0.481 pmpm

- The estimated overhead costs required to support the management of the contract (See Section J for a detailed discussion of the management requirements), expressed as a PMPM number.

- The estimated profit for the psychiatric practice, expressed as a PMPM number.

G. Cost of Clinical Services

The cost of clinical services is one component of the capitation rate. It expresses the psychiatric practice's projection of the cost of delivering direct clinical services to the covered group and results from the following formula:

Cost of Service $=$ Number of Services $\times$ Cost per Unit of Service

H. Estimating the Number of Services

Estimating the number of services to be delivered is a function of the following variables:

Population penetration—Number of covered members who will seek services expressed as a percentage of the entire covered group.

Utilization per 1,000—Number of services used by the covered members expressed per 1,000 lives. This number is derived by calculating the total episodes of care, the average length of each episode, and the total number of units of service.

The formula for services per 1,000 lives may be used to calculate the statistic for any time period chosen, such as for the day, the month, year to date, and so forth. When calculating bed days per 1,000, use the assumption of a 365-day year as opposed to a 12-month year to prevent variations that are due solely to the length of the month.[5] The

---

[5] Kongstvedt, P. "Controlling Hospital Utilization," *The Managed Healthcare Handbook*, 1993, page 103.

III

formula, which is for illustrative purposes only, is as follows (see also Figure 2):

$$[A \div (B \div 365)] \div C \div 1,000)$$

A = services per time unit
B = days per time unit
C = plan membership

This calculation should be made for hospital days, outpatient visits, and all other levels of care included under the contract.

Depending upon the types of covered services as defined in the benefit plan, the psychiatric practice must determine the utilization of services for a variety of levels of care. A common "continuum of care" for which utilization may need to be projected, depending on the terms of the contract, is as follows:

Inpatient Hospitalization
Partial Hospitalization and Day Treatment
Residential Services
Intensive Outpatient Services
Outpatient Services

Again, depending upon the benefit plan, these utilization projections should be separately calculated for both mental health and chemical dependency services. Also, given the psychiatric practice's scope of

---

FIGURE 2 **Sample Calculation for Days per 1,000 for a Month**

ASSUME: Total bed days in month = 300 (A)
Days in month = 31 (B)
Plan membership = 12,000 (C)

Step 1: Gross days month to date
= A ÷ (B ÷ 365)
= 300 ÷ (31 ÷ 365)
= 300 ÷ 0.08493
= 3,532.32

Step 2: Days per 1,000 in month
= Result of Step 1 ÷ (C ÷ 1,000)
= 3,532.32 ÷ (12,000 ÷ 1,000)
= 3,532.32 ÷ 12
= 294.36 days per 1,000

practice or the composition of the network, this continuum may be expanded or contracted to reflect the range of services available for member treatment.

Combining these variables into an experience table for a member group of 92,000 covered lives for one year of service might look like that shown in Table 8.

I. Estimating the Cost per Unit of Service

Combining the utilization projections with the cost of service estimates will yield the first round of the capitation rate. Costs for services can be determined as follows:

- If the psychiatric group is accepting capitation for its services only, a full cost study should be completed to determine both the direct and indirect costs for each type of service to be delivered by the psychiatric practice under the capitation arrangement. This can be derived from the practice's financial and statistical reports, and it should take into account all of the overhead expenses required to deliver those services.

Sample Utilization by Level of Care

TABLE 8

Level of Care	% of Covered Population Using Services	Admits	Average Length of Stay	Total Units	Days/Visits per 1,000
Inpatient MH	0.324%	298	6.8	2,013	21.9
Partial MH	0.070%	65	6.4	412	4.5
Alternative Res. MH	0.002%	2	155.3	278	3.0
Outpatient MH	1.666%	1,533	6.8	10,420	113.3
Inpatient CD	0.064%	59	6.2	366	4.0
Partial CD	0.038%	35	6.8	237	2.6
Alternative Res. CD	0.003%	2	8.5	20	0.2
Outpatient CD	0.006%	6	4.2	25	0.3

III

- If the psychiatric practice is providing services through a network of psychiatrists who are not a part of the practice, then the psychiatric practice should have contracts with those psychiatrists who state the rates to be paid for various services. If these psychiatrists include hospital units and other facility-based services, then per diem contracts should be obtained to facilitate cost projections, as well as to contain costs for the contract.

The determination of unit costs can be fairly straightforward for institutional services based on per diem payments. If, for example, the psychiatric inpatient service network consists of two hospitals, one with a $400 per diem and the other with a $500 per diem, a simple average or weighted average based on the projected volume of services to be delivered by each can be used. Table 9 is an example.

A similar method can be used to determine the average cost per unit of outpatient service when the psychiatric group uses clinicians with varying disciplines and contract rates. Table 10 is an example.

TABLE 9

Weighted Average Cost per Day

Facility	Total Days	Per Diem	Total Cost
Unit A	250	$400	$100,000
Unit B	350	$500	$175,000
Totals	600		$275,000
		Weighted Average Cost per Day	$458.33

TABLE 10

Weighted Average Cost per Visit

Psychiatrist Discipline	Total Visits	Per Visit	Total Cost
Psychiatrists	3,500	$100	$350,000
Psychologists	1,350	$80	$108,000
Social Workers	3,000	$70	$210,000
Totals	7,850		$668,000
		Weighted Average Cost per Visit	$85.10

As evident in Table 10, varying the "mix" of psychiatric disciplines can have a substantial effect on the average cost per visit. For this reason, many psychiatrists strive to use lower-cost disciplines for routine procedures in a capitated environment. This strategy allows the psychiatric practice to better manage the costs for these services, and it also frees valuable time to focus on the difficult, high-cost cases that are sure to emerge when providing services to a large group.

J. Estimating Overhead Costs

Every capitated arrangement will require support services and an administrative infrastructure to support the services directly provided by the psychiatric practice and to support the authorization and payment of services provided by others through a network. These overhead costs should be carefully detailed and added to the direct costs of clinical services to arrive at an equitable capitation rate for the psychiatric practice. Failure to incorporate some portion of overhead costs in a capitated arrangement can lead to negative financial results for the psychiatric practice.

Overhead costs can be estimated by preparing a budget outlining the type, number, and costs of the services required to support management of the contract. The total cost of these administrative services is then converted into a PMPM rate and added to the direct clinical cost PMPM to continue building the capitation estimate.

An example of a typical overhead calculation for a 92,000 member group is shown in Table 11. (Please note that the staff and costs are illustrative only and should not be interpreted as a recommended sizing for an administrative infrastructure for a capitated contract.)

Some of the elements influencing the type and size of supporting administrative infrastructure are as follows:

- Type of clinical management protocol utilized;

- Number of covered lives and number of benefit plans administered;

III

- Use and required size of a psychiatrist network;

- Quality and clinical efficiency of the psychiatric practice and/or the psychiatric practice network;

- National Committee on Quality Assurance (NCQA) and Health Plan Employer Data and Information Set (HEDIS) reporting requirements;

- Need to upgrade computer system;

- Presence and nature of claims payment requirements; and

- Presence and nature of member service requirements.

As with utilization control and risk management, a large group allows the psychiatric practice to more effectively spread the overhead costs.

TABLE 11	**Sample Overhead Costs With 92,000 Covered Members**		
Item	**Units Required**	**Cost per Month***	**Total Cost**
Director of Clinical Services	1.0 FTE	$5,417	$65,000
Executive Medical Director	0.5 FTE	7,292	87,500
Case Management Staff	3.0 FTE	11,250	135,000
Secretarial Staff	2.0 FTE	4,167	50,000
Psychiatrist Relations Staff	1.0 FTE	2,917	35,000
Finance Staff	1.0 FTE	2,917	35,000
Claims Processing Staff	2.0 FTE	4,167	50,000
Member Services Staff	2.0 FTE	4,167	50,000
Information Systems Staff	1.0 FTE	2,917	35,000
Sales and Marketing Staff	0.5 FTE	1,875	22,500
Rent and Utilities	n/a	4,000	48,000
Telephone System	n/a	2,000	24,000
Other Overhead	n/a	3,000	36,000
		Total Overhead Costs	$673,000
Per Member per Month ($673,000/12/92,000)			$0.610

*Numbers have been rounded.

Further, if overhead costs can be allocated among several different capitation contracts, the psychiatric practice can allocate more of each capitation rate to clinical service delivery and profit.

K.   Profit and Capital Allowances

The third major component of a capitation rate (the first is clinical service costs, the second is overhead costs) is the allocation of an amount for profit and an allowance for capital costs. This can be either a fixed cost added to the two other components of clinical service costs and overhead or a percentage of the total costs. The latter method is the most common. Although there is wide variation in the percentage of profit allocated to a contract, a common range is 6% to 10% of total costs.

L.   Sample Capitation Rate Calculation

Calculating a capitation rate is a six-step process.

L.1.   Step One: Determine the Benefit Plan and Member Group

This example uses the following assumptions:

- The benefit is a traditional HMO plan with coverage for both mental health and chemical dependency services.

- There is an annual combined limit of 20 outpatient visits and 30 inpatient days.

- There is a $10 copayment per outpatient visit and a $25 copayment per inpatient day. There is no deductible or out-of-pocket maximum for the covered member or the family.

- All services must be delivered by a network practitioner, and all services must be pre-authorized by the psychiatric group.

- The covered group is a mixture of commercial HMO patient companies with a total of 35,000 covered lives.

III

L.2. Step Two: Determine the Utilization Rates for the Group

Based on experience data provided by the plan and the psychiatric practice's estimate of the impact its clinical management will produce, the utilization projections shown in Table 12 were established (the table is for illustration purposes only).

L.3. Step Three: Determine the Costs of Services

The psychiatric group will use a network of clinicians and facilities to augment services provided by the group. They have contracted with a sufficient number of external resources, and they use fee schedules and per diems in their contracting. Table 13 lists the average costs per unit of service.

The outpatient mental health cost was derived using a weighted average among disciplines in the network. In order to contain costs and utilize valuable psychiatrist time in management of more difficult cases, the group elected to use lower-cost disciplines to deliver routine outpatient care.

Once the unit costs are determined, the next step is to apply these costs to the projected utilization, as demonstrated in Table 14.

TABLE 12

Sample Utilization Projections

Level of Care	% of Covered Population Using Services	Admits	Average Length of Stay	Totals	Days/Visits per 1,000
Inpatient MH	0.267%	93	11.6	1,083	30.9
Partial MH	0.120%	42	6.4	269	7.7
Alternative Res. MH	0.000%	0	0.0	0	0
Outpatient MH	3.831%	1,341	8.7	11,725	335
Inpatient CD	0.010%	4	13.0	48	1.4
Partial CD	0.005%	2	5.0	9	0.3
Alternative Res. CD	0.010%	4	11.0	40	1.2
Outpatient CD	0.016%	5	3.0	16	0.5

III

The formulas for the cells in Table 14 are as follows:

$$\text{Total Costs} = \text{Units per 1,000} \times \text{Unit Cost}$$
$$\text{Cost PMPM} = \text{Total Costs} \div 12 \div 1,000$$

After developing the gross costs of care projected for this population, the next step is to calculate the value of the benefit plan's copayment and deductible provisions. These are converted into PMPM numbers and deducted from the gross cost of care (see Table 15).

Average Cost per Unit of Service

TABLE 13

Level of Care	Cost per Unit
Inpatient MH	$450 per day
Partial MH	$200 per day
Alternative Res. MH	$50 per day
Outpatient MH	$75 per visit
Inpatient CD	$450 per day
Partial CD	$200 per day
Alternative Res. CD	$50 per day
Outpatient CD	$75 per visit

Costs Based on Utilization Projections

TABLE 14

Level of Care	Days/Visits per 1,000	Unit Costs	Total Costs	Cost PMPM
Inpatient MH	30.9	$450	$13,905	$1.159
Partial MH	7.7	200	1,540	0.128
Alternative Res. MH	0	50	0	0
Outpatient MH	335	75	25,125	2.094
Inpatient CD	1.4	450	630	0.053
Partial CD	0.3	200	60	0.005
Alternative Res. CD	1.2	50	60	0.005
Outpatient CD	0.5	75	37.50	0.003
		Total Costs	$41,357.50	$3.447

III

Deducting the copayment revenue from the gross cost of services yields the net cost of clinical care (see Table 16).

One factor for the psychiatric group to consider is that the revenue from copayments represents income to the practice if the practice is providing the service and collecting the copayments from the members. However, co-pays are more risky than collecting all fees from an MCO (must assume some bad debt) and have costs associated with

TABLE 15

Revenue From Copayments

Level of Care	Plan Copayment	Utilization	Resulting Revenue
Inpatient MH	$25 per day	1,083	$27,705
Partial MH	none	269	0
Alternative Res. MH	none	0	0
Outpatient MH	$10 per visit	11,725	117,250
Inpatient CD	$25 per day	48	1,200
Partial CD	none	9	0
Alternative Res. CD	none	40	0
Outpatient CD	$10 per visit	16	160

TABLE 16

Net Cost per Member per Month

Level of Care	Total Costs	Copayment Revenue	Net Cost of Care	Net Cost PMPM
Inpatient MH	$487,350	$27,705	$459,645	$1.094
Partial MH	53,800	0	53,800	0.128
Alternative Res. MH	0	0	0	0
Outpatient MH	879,375	117,250	762,125	1.814
Inpatient CD	21,600	1,200	20,400	0.049
Partial CD	1,800	0	0	0.004
Alternative Res. CD	2,000	0	0	0.005
Outpatient CD	1,200	160	1,040	0.002
Total Costs	$1,447,125	$146,315	$1,297,010	$3.098

them (collections). This expense should be deducted from the expected revenue of the practice when calculating the projected capitation rate.

L.4. Step Four: Determine the Costs of Overhead Requirements

Adjusting the overhead costs illustrated earlier to a sample size of 35,000 covered lives, the psychiatric group estimates the overhead requirements for this contract to be those shown in Table 17.

In completing Table 17, there are several considerations:

- The categories listed are not meant to be exclusive. Additional items should be added that will affect the psychiatric practice's ability to manage the capitation contract. These may include costs such as information systems acquisition or access costs; costs of

Sample Overhead Costs With 35,000 Covered Lives

TABLE 17

Item	Units Required	Cost per Month	Total Cost
Director of Clinical Services	0.5 FTE	$2,708	$32,500
Executive Medical Director	0.25 FTE	3,646	43,750
Case Management Staff	1.0 FTE	3,750	45,000
Secretarial Staff	1.0 FTE	2,083	25,000
Psychiatrist Relations Staff	1.0 FTE	2,917	35,000
Finance Staff	1.0 FTE	2,917	35,000
Claims Processing Staff	1.0 FTE	2,083	25,000
Member Services Staff	1.0 FTE	2,083	25,000
Information Systems Staff	0.5 FTE	1,458	17,500
Sales and Marketing Staff	0.5 FTE	1,875	22,500
Rent and Utilities	n/a	2,000	24,000
Telephone System	n/a	1,000	12,000
Other Overhead	n/a	2,000	24,000
		Total Overhead Costs	$366,250
	Per Member per Month ($366,250/12/35,000)		$0.872

III

licenses and certifications required for risk arrangements in the psychiatrist's state; consultation costs, including legal, actuarial, programmatic, and clinical; peer review costs for those cases going outside of the psychiatrist's practice; the cost of stop-loss insurance or other reinsurance mechanisms; quality improvement staff and associated costs; and charges for other services necessary for the adequate management of the contract and the patients receiving treatment.

- Depending upon the accounting practices of the psychiatric practice, the relative length of the contract, and/or the presence of other capitation contracts, the practice may choose to amortize certain overhead costs over an extended period or to allocate fixed overhead expenses across a number of capitation contracts, with the allocation method being based on the ratio of contract covered lives to total covered lives; the ratio of contract claims expenses to total claims expenses; or a time-based or activity-based formula.

- As a rule of thumb, conventional capitation contracts usually target total overhead and profit amounts to no more than 15% of the premium (the remaining 85% is allocated to the cost of care and is referred to as the "loss ratio").

There is a valid argument that mental health capitation rates may include an overhead/profit percentage in excess of 15%. This is due to the following factors:

- There is a vast difference between a full medical/surgical premium and the relatively small mental health capitation amount. For example, an average premium yield for a medical/surgical capitation may approach $125 PMPM. Of this amount, 15% yields $18.75 per member per month for overhead and profit; 15% of a typical mental health capitation of $3.25 per member per month yields only $0.4875 per member per month for overhead and profit.

- However, many mental health capitation arrangements require the capitated mental health practice to have the same infrastructure as the medical/surgical MCO, such as claims, member services, case management, provider relations, marketing, and information systems. Although the mental health management requirements are substantially less than that for a medical/surgical MCO (generally about 10% of the typical medical/surgical MCO), there is a certain baseline level of infrastructure and fixed costs that drive up the percentage of the capitation allocated to these costs. Given this, it is not unusual to find overhead and profit percentages of up to 30% to 35% in mental health capitation calculations.

Before an allocation for profit and capital costs, the capitation rate now equals the following:

Direct Cost of Care	$3.098
Overhead Costs	$0.872
Total Rate	$3.970

L.5. Step Five: Determine the Profit Expectation

Using a standard percentage of total costs of 6%, the per member per month profit allocation would equal the following:

Direct Cost of Care	$3.098
Overhead Costs	$0.872
Profit at 6%	$0.238
Preliminary Rate	$4.208

L.6. Step Six: Test For Reasonableness

As recommended earlier, the preliminary rate and the estimates upon which it is based should be developed in concert with an actuary familiar with mental health capitation strategies and data. Once the preliminary rate has been developed, it is helpful to "test" the rate against known benchmarks and an estimate of the prevailing market rates for similar services. A useful tool is the *Capitation Handbook,* developed for the American Psychiatric Association (APA) by Milliman and Robertson, Inc., an actuarial and consulting firm. Published in 1995, the handbook gives an excellent overview of the basics of capita-

III

tion and capitation contracting. More importantly, the handbook contains a variety of capitation rates for different plan designs and member populations. As such, it can serve as a useful comparative instrument with which to judge the reasonableness of a mental health capitation estimate.

Using the handbook's capitation estimates for a commercial population produces the following comparisons: the rates for a similar benefit plan for a commercial population range from $4.27 to $6.11 for a moderately managed plan.

Although the benefit plan used for comparison differed in that it accounted for higher copayments and deductibles, the preliminary rate calculated above seems to compare favorably.

Additional comparisons using local market rates are also of use in determining the reasonableness of capitation rate calculations. In the event that the calculated rate does not compare favorably, i.e., it is substantially higher than benchmarks or local market rates, the psychiatric group has the following options in assessing its rate assumptions:

- Review the utilization assumptions and determine the effect of tighter clinical management controls and the practice's ability to accomplish this.

- Review the unit cost assumptions and determine if improvements in rates can be obtained through better contract negotiation and/ or use of lower-cost psychiatrists.

- Review the overhead cost assumptions to determine if a lower allocation is feasible, while retaining the capability to manage the contract and recoup costs.

- Review the profit and capital allocation to determine if lower rates are possible.

If the practice is unable to modify these factors and negotiate an equitable rate that is consistent with prevailing market rates and the payer's expectations, a re-evaluation of the practice's capability or

III

desire to enter into these kinds of arrangements is in order. It must be stated that there are market conditions in which extremely low capitation rate expectations prevail, and in the words of a psychiatrist experienced in these matters, "I can manage care at those rates; I just don't choose to."

Evaluating and Negotiating a Capitation Contract

A psychiatrist evaluating a capitated contract should consider the proposed capitation rate and the operational terms of the contract.

A. Assessment of the Proposed Capitation Rate

The psychiatric practice, with the assistance of an actuary, should review the proposed capitation rate and evaluate the following assumptions for reasonableness and the psychiatric practice's ability to deliver the care required under those assumptions.

Population Penetration

- Is the number of members that are projected to require services consistent with the history of the group?

- Does the psychiatric practice have prior experience with this group and the management techniques used in the past?

- What is the penetration by level of care? Is there a disproportionate number of members receiving care at high levels of intensity (i.e., inpatient)?

- Can the psychiatric practice implement clinical management measures to favorably impact the number of members presenting for care? What are those measures and what will the likely impact be?

IV

Episodes of Care

■　What is the average length of stay allocated to each level of care? Are the lengths of stay reasonable?

■　Can the psychiatric practice implement contracting and clinical management measures to favorably impact the length of stay? For example, can the psychiatric practice increase the range of services to include more effective, less intensive levels of care? What are those measures and what will the likely impact be?

Overhead Allocations

■　What are the assumptions used in allocating the overhead expenses? Are they reasonable?

■　Can the psychiatric practice make improvements in the administration of the contract to meet the overhead targets?

Profit and Capital Allowances

■　What are the assumptions for profit and capital, and how were they applied to the rate? Are they reasonable?

B.　　Operational Terms of the Contract

There are a variety of assessments the psychiatric practice can make to determine if the terms of the contract are reasonable. They fall into four major groups: payment provisions, duties of the psychiatric practice, duties of the MCO, and general provisions.

B.1.　　Payment Provisions

The services covered under the capitation agreement should be clearly defined. The contract should also state services or procedures that are *not* covered by the agreement. Also, the geographic area covered by the agreement should be clearly delineated.

The psychiatric practice and actuary should carefully assess any stop-loss or risk corridor provisions of the contract to determine the potential impact on the ultimate risk assumed by the practice. A sample calculation should be verified by the plan so that the psychiatric practice clearly understands the amount and nature of the risk protection being offered. The cost of any stop-loss provisions also should be clearly defined.

The payment provisions of the contract should clearly state the definition of an "eligible member" along with the responsibility of the psychiatric practice for determining eligibility at the time of service. Also, the contract should clearly state how and when the capitation will be paid and upon what membership count the total payment will be based. A typical clause for this section of the contract is as follows:

> *Compensation to psychiatrist for Capitated Services shall be a fixed monthly prepayment referred to as "Capitation." Payment to the psychiatric practice shall be made by the 10th day of the month for all members eligible to receive services at the 1st of the month. In the event an HMO Member is not eligible to receive services during the entire month, the capitation payment for that Member-month shall be prorated to the number of days the Member will be eligible.*

Equally important is the provision that allows for a reconciliation of the capitation payment at the end of the contract year to account for members enrolling and disenrolling in the middle of a month.

Another contract provision to assess is the treatment of patient copayments and deductibles, referred to as "patient cost-sharing." Generally, the psychiatric practice is entitled to the collection of copayments and deductibles for patients receiving services. The contract should state how this revenue is treated in the calculation of the capitation rate. If the projected value of the copayments and deductibles are deducted from the capitation rate, the contract should be clear about the psychiatric practice's responsibility to deliver services to those members who cannot or refuse to pay the cost-sharing provision.

The psychiatric practice should also examine the contract provisions for its rights and responsibilities in the event of a default by the plan.

Finally, the psychiatric practice should understand the provisions of the contract regarding the coordination of benefits (COB) for those

members with secondary coverage by another plan. The psychiatric
practice should clearly understand its obligations in this regard.

B.2.   Duties of the Psychiatric Practice

This section of the contract should clearly define the responsibilities of
the psychiatric practice in several important areas:

Medical records What are the plan's access rights to medical records?
Who obtains patient consent to release records?

Credentialing What credentialing material should the psychiatric practice maintain personally and for contracted participants in its group
or network? Will the psychiatric practice have to meet NCQA guidelines in this respect?

Contracting What contractual arrangements can the psychiatric practice employ for participants in its practice or network? Are there
any restrictions on risk transfer to other psychiatrists or psychiatric
practices (i.e., subcapitation, case rates, withholds, etc.)? What oversight does the plan have over the psychiatric practice or network?
Does the plan have the right to preclude certain psychiatrists from
participation? Does the plan have the right to publish the names of
those in the psychiatric practice's network in materials distributed to
members?

Member services Does the contract define specific appeals and grievance procedures for members? If the plan has the final authority in
appeals, what is the mechanism employed by the plan in exercising
that authority? Does the psychiatric practice have any responsibilities
for communicating with members or assisting the plan in its member
recruitment and marketing activities?

Utilization review What are the provisions for utilization review in the
contract? Do all services have to be pre-authorized before the psychiatric practice is liable for delivery and/or payment?

What are the definitions of "medical necessity" and "emergency care"?

Does the psychiatric practice have to meet NCQA process and reporting requirements in this area? Is any other certification or license required by the plan?

What is the role of primary care physicians (PCPs) in the authorization process? Do members have to receive an authorization/referral from the PCP before accessing care by the psychiatric practice?

What are the contractual provisions for patients who refuse to comply with treatment?

What are the provisions for "out-of-area" care? Is the cost of these services the responsibility of the psychiatric practice under the capitation? If so, what is the cost basis for payment of such care (i.e., payment equivalent to the average contracted cost, usual and customary charges, etc.)?

What is the process for determining cost liability for members with concurrent psychiatric and physical diagnoses? What are the provisions for payment of medically necessary services delivered by a non-psychiatrist (i.e., a PCP, pediatrician, internist, etc.)? How are consultations handled and cost-accounted? How are claims handled?

If the plan covers an employer with an employee assistance program (EAP), what is the role of the EAP in service authorization?

Reporting What kinds of reports are required by the plan? What are the format and frequency of these reports? Are there penalty provisions for failure to provide timely reports?

Quality assurance What are the quality assurance responsibilities of the psychiatric practice? Does the psychiatric practice have to meet NCQA process and reporting requirements in this area?

B.3.   Duties of the MCO
The contract should contain provisions defining the duties of the MCO under capitation. Specific areas for assessment are as follows:

Membership What are the responsibilities of the plan regarding the provision of membership eligibility data to the psychiatric practice?

How will this be accomplished, and what medium will be used (i.e., paper lists, telephone contact with the plan, electronic data exchange, online access to the plan's information system, etc.)?

What are the provisions of the contract in the event the plan makes errors in eligibility? Specifically, what are the remedies to the psychiatric practice if services are delivered to a member who later is determined to be ineligible for coverage?

Will the psychiatric practice have to meet NCQA reporting requirements in this area? On what system will "continuous enrollment" data be based?

Will the plan be required to pay the psychiatric practice by a specific date each month for each enrollee who chooses or is assigned to the psychiatric practice for that month?

Does the agreement identify the covered services that the psychiatric practice is required to provide for the capitated payment?

Marketing How will the name of the practice and/or network be used in plan marketing activities? Does the psychiatric practice have the right to inspect and approve any marketing materials in this area?

Appeals What are the plan's rights and responsibilities in the appeal and grievance process? Who are the members of the plan's appeals committee, and what is the psychiatric practice's role in interacting with that committee?

B.4. General Provisions

Indemnification Are there provisions requiring the psychiatric practice to indemnify the plan? The psychiatric practice may wish to negotiate a provision for a low-enrollment guarantee. (For example, compensation will be provided on a fee-for-service basis until a certain minimum enrollment is achieved.)

Termination What are the termination provisions of the contract? Specifically, what are the psychiatric practice's duties for patients in treatment during and after the cancellation period? Is there a provision

for contract termination without cause by either party? What are the
notification time lines and requirements in the event of a termination?

Coverage What specific groups and members does this contract cover?
Are new groups and new contracts acquired by the plan included in
the capitation agreement? What is the process for notifying the psychiatric practice of new groups?

Confidentiality What are the provisions for patient confidentiality in
the agreement?

C.   Understanding Benefit Exclusions

Equally important as the definition of covered services is the definition
of services not covered by the capitation agreement.

Below is a listing of typical non-covered services.

- Tobacco dependence, tics and sleep disorders, frontal lobe syndrome, and specific delays in development;

- Services that are extended beyond the period necessary for the
  evaluation and diagnosis of mental retardation, developmental
  disabilities, and/or autism;

- Any services for speech therapy, remedial education diagnosis and
  treatment, weight loss, and personal growth;

- Treatment of chronic pain, other than by psychotherapy if such
  pain is determined to be of psychological origin;

- Rehabilitative treatment associated with hearing and/or vision
  impairment, or rehabilitative treatment associated with permanent
  or temporary disability resulting from an accident or injury in
  circumstances where such treatment is part of a comprehensive
  rehabilitative program;

- Treatments that are considered to be experimental and unproven
  and/or treatments that are research protocol–driven including,
  but not limited to, drug trials, psychosurgery, megavitamin ther-

IV

apy, nutritionally based therapies for alcoholism and substance abuse, non-abstinence-based substance abuse treatments, and codependency;

- Any consultations, interventions, or ongoing medical services provided by non-licensed psychiatric physicians or non-physician practitioners for conditions, disorders, and/or complications not directly related to the diagnosis and/or treatment of a primary mental illness;

- Psychiatric or psychological examinations, testing, or treatments for purposes of obtaining or maintaining employment or insurance or relating to judicial or administrative proceedings or for educational purposes;

- Treatment for mental illness and/or substance abuse when required by an order of court of competent jurisdiction when such an order is made without the knowledge of the psychiatric practice or is inconsistent with the psychiatric practice's assessment and recommendation for treatment, including orders of probation or parole as an alternative to same;

- Treatment in institutions for chronic and/or rehabilitative care;

- Treatment of organic brain syndrome, Alzheimer's disease, senile dementia, or AIDS dementia; and

- Pharmaceutical agents or the costs of laboratory testing for the side effects of pharmaceutical agents.

A contract attachment should be developed by the psychiatric practice and the plan outlining service exclusions similar to that presented above.

D.   Dispute Resolution and/or Procedures for "Gray Area" Services

The negotiation of the contract should also include provisions for the resolution of disputes relating to services delivered for patients with concurrent psychiatric and physical diagnoses and for medically necessary services delivered by non-psychiatric physicians. For example, a clear understanding of the responsibility of the psychiatric practice should be obtained for attention-deficit/hyperactivity disorder treatment services delivered by a pediatrician. Another example is the provision by a PCP of psychopharmaceuticals to a depressed patient. See Appendix 1 for an example of policy guidelines typically used for determination of liability in cases such as these.

E.   Checklist for Evaluating Capitated Agreements

Following is a contract checklist for evaluating a capitated agreement. The checklist details those important contract provisions and issues that should be reviewed and analyzed before entering into a capitation contract.

E.1.   Introductory Contract Provisions
Identification of Parties

- Are the parties to the contract properly identified?

- Are all affiliates of the HMO who are also bound to the contract clearly identified?

- Is the legal status of the psychiatric entity or individual psychiatrist clearly stated?

Recitals/Whereas Clauses

- Are the recitals or whereas clauses clear, and do they represent the understanding of the parties to the agreement? *(The recitals or whereas clauses should not attempt to expand the scope of the contract beyond its own terms.)*

Definitions

- Does the contract contain a definitions section that clearly sets forth the parties' understanding of the scope of each term? *(This section should, at a minimum, contain detailed definitions of the*

IV

terms "Member" or "Enrollee" and "Capitated Services" and/or
"Covered Services.")

E.2.   Compensation

Capitation Payment Rates

- Is the psychiatric practice receiving capitation in the form of a percentage of monthly member premiums?

- Receiving a PMPM payment rate?

- Is the psychiatric practice capable of accepting capitation?

- Does the psychiatric practice need minimum member enrollment requirements or minimum fee-for-service payment equivalent levels before accepting capitation?

Copayments and Deductibles

- Does the contract allow psychiatrists to directly collect copayments and deductibles from members and pursue members for nonpayment?

Capitated Services

- Does the contract specify which services are Capitated Services for which the psychiatric practice shall receive a monthly capitation payment, and which services are Covered Services that include non-Capitated Services?

"Carve-Out" Services

- Does the contract or an attachment detail certain Covered Services that are "carved-out" of capitation and paid on a fee-for-service basis?

Stop-Loss Provisions

- Does the contract include stop-loss protection or provide for reinsurance?

- Is the threshold for stop-loss/reinsurance reasonable?

- What is the psychiatric practice's required contribution?

- Is reinsurance available from outside sources?

Rate Renegotiation

- How often will rates be renegotiated?

- Can the psychiatric practice request a renegotiated rate based on changes in plan design or member selection factors?

E.3. Psychiatrist Duties

Network Requirements

- Does the psychiatric practice have to have a certain network composition in place?

- Specifically, are certain psychiatrists or types of psychiatrists required by the contract?

- Are there time and geographic access requirements for the network?

Performance Standards

- Are there any performance standards in the contract?

- Specifically, are there standards related to access such as minimum waiting times for appointments, access by telephone to a clinician, minimum hold times on the telephone, etc.?

- Are there standards related to utilization such as minimum utilization levels?

- Are there standards for administrative operations such as claim processing times, appeal processing times, etc.?

- Are there any financial penalties or rewards associated with these standards?

Management Reports

- What types of reports are required by the HMO?

- Are there templates and due dates for the reports?

- Will the psychiatric practice have to provide NCQA- and HEDIS-compliant reports?

- Are there penalties for failure to provide the reports in a timely fashion?

Provision of Services

- Does the contract clearly explain the duties of the psychiatric practice?

- Does the contract have a detailed list of actual covered services in a separate attachment to the contract?

- Does the contract provide procedures for referral of members to other psychiatrists for certain services?

Maintenance of Standards

- Does the contract explain the required standards and licensure requirements that the psychiatric practice must maintain?

- Are the standards reasonable within the local medical community?

- Is the group practice obligated to ensure performance by its contracting individual psychiatrists?

Participation in Utilization Review and Quality Improvement Activities

- Does the contract specify responsibilities of the psychiatric practice in connection with quality improvement (QI) and utilization review (UR) activities?

- Will the psychiatric practice have to participate on any QI/UR committees established by the HMO?

- Will the psychiatric practice have to establish internal QI/UR mechanisms?

- Will the psychiatric practice have to assist the HMO in meeting NCQA standards?

Maintenance of Insurance

- Does the contract require the psychiatric practice to maintain general liability and professional liability coverage?

- Does the psychiatric practice's coverage meet the HMO's requested coverage limits?

- Does the group practice have an insurance obligation separate from its contracting individual psychiatrists?

- Must the HMO maintain insurance?

Encounter Data and Billing

- Does the contract contain a provision requiring psychiatrists to maintain information regarding member utilization of services?

- Does the contract specify under what circumstances a psychiatrist may bill a patient for services?

Patient "Hold Harmless" Provision

- Does the contract contain a section prohibiting the psychiatric practice from pursuing patients directly for payment for Covered Services?

- Does it still allow psychiatrists to collect copayments and deductibles and fees for non-Covered Services?

Continuation of Services

- Does the contract provide for the continuation of services by a psychiatrist after termination of the contract?

- For how long?

- Is the period reasonable?

- How is the psychiatric practice compensated during the continuation period?

IV

Medicare and Medicaid Programs

- Does the contract state that psychiatrists will provide services to Medicare/Medicaid members?

- Are methods of compensation and stop-loss/risk-pool arrangements separate from commercial compensation?

- Is the psychiatric practice required to be Medicaid/Medicare certified?

- Is the psychiatric practice capable of providing a full range of required Medicare/Medicaid services?

E.4.   MCO Duties
Administration

- Are administrative responsibilities of the MCO stated?

Eligibility Information

- How often will the MCO give its psychiatrists updated eligibility information/lists?

- Can psychiatrists rely upon the list when deciding whether or not to provide Covered Services to someone?

- Who is responsible for errors in information on lists?

Provision of Necessary Data

- What information will the HMO give to its psychiatrists regarding the HMO's health plans?

- To its members?

Payments to Psychiatrists

- Is there a specific provision in the body of the contract indicating how and when payment will be made to psychiatrists?

- Is it explained in an attachment to the contract?

E.5.   Other Considerations

Coordination of Benefits

- Does the HMO contract impose any collection duties on psychiatrists when an HMO is coordinating benefits?

Exclusivity of Relationships

- Does the contract provide for an exclusive relationship between the HMO and the psychiatric practice?

- Is consideration provided in exchange for a psychiatrist agreeing to work exclusively with the HMO?

- Are both parties agreeing to exclusivity?

Terms of the Contract

- What is the effective date of the contract?

- How long is the term of the contract?

- Does it automatically renew or do the parties have to enter into a new contract upon its expiration?

Termination of the Contract

- Does the contract provide for termination without cause?

- By both parties?

- Does the contract provide for termination with cause?

- By both parties?

- Does contract define the term "material cause," which may give rise to termination?

- Is there a cure period before the contract is terminated with cause?

- Must the psychiatric practice continue to provide Covered Services after the contract is terminated?

IV

Indemnification

- Does the contract provide for mutual indemnification?

- For indemnification only by the psychiatric practice?

- Does it extend the indemnification beyond the scope of a party's insurance coverage?

Confidentiality of Medical Records

- Does the contract provide for the confidential maintenance of member medical records by both the psychiatric practice and the MCO?

Audit of Financial Records

- Does the contract allow the psychiatric practice to audit the financial records of an MCO to determine whether or not he or she is receiving appropriate capitation payments?

Member Transfers

- Does the contract allow the psychiatric practice to request the transfer of a member who is disruptive/refusing treatment?

- Can the MCO unilaterally transfer members away from a psychiatrist at any time?

E.6. Boilerplate Language
Amendments

- Is the MCO able to amend the contract if there are changes in relevant state/federal laws or regulations?

- Can the MCO unilaterally amend the contract?

- Is the psychiatric practice able to object to some amendments, including changes to the MCO's psychiatrist manual?

- Can parties amend the contract by mutual agreement?

Assignment

- Does the contract provide for mutual assignment or assignment only by the MCO?

Dispute Resolution

- Can the parties utilize informal procedures to resolve disputes?

- Is arbitration or mediation the parties' final recourse?

- Can the parties adopt their own rules or must they follow the rules of the American Arbitration Association?

Other Documents Incorporated by Reference

- Does the contract reference other documents to which the parties are bound, such as psychiatrist manuals, MCO policies and procedures manuals, and patient materials and contracts?

- Are documents available for review prior to execution of the contract with the MCO?

Generally, mental health capitation contracts provide for an initial contract term of two or more years. The parties usually want to lock each other into a longer term of contract because they have taken the time to negotiate a contract that contains terms and compensation rates that the parties have mutually agreed upon. Upon expiration of the initial contract term, the contract will usually provide for automatic renewal on the anniversary of the expiration of the initial term of the contract.

If the term provision of a contract provides for automatic renewal of the contract upon the expiration of each successive term, the contract will not expire until one of the parties provides notice of termination to the other. In addition, unless the contract provides for amendment of the contract terms by either party, the terms negotiated for the initial term of the contract will remain in effect throughout each renewal of the contract.

Organizational and Administrative Issues in Managing a Capitated Contract

Some of the factors determining the size and scope of the administrative infrastructure for a capitated psychiatric practice include the following:

- Type of clinical management protocol utilized;

- Number of covered lives and number of benefit plans administered;

- Use and required size of a psychiatrist network;

- Quality and clinical efficiency of the psychiatric practice and/or the psychiatric practice network;

- NCQA and HEDIS reporting requirements;

- Presence and nature of claims payment requirements; and

- Presence and nature of member service requirements.

A. Clinical Management Issues

In order to succeed in a capitated arrangement, the psychiatric practice must have the following clinical management system capabilities:

- Coordinated and standardized core clinical processes, such as dedicated points of access and referral for the member requesting services;

- Clinical oversight and monitoring mechanisms, such as clinical case management protocols and utilization review procedures;

- For comprehensive capitation contracts, an expansive continuum of service delivery that is community-based. This might include a range of outpatient and crisis intervention programs and home-based and community residential alternatives for certain member populations, such as Medicaid patients.

- Clinical pathways (charts that show key events leading to the successful treatment of patients in a certain homogenous population) and practice guidelines (standards of treatment for specific illnesses) that facilitate standardization of care and permit the profiling and tracking of psychiatrist performance and patient progress. The APA has available a series of publications about practice guidelines. The price for each guideline publication is $22.50, as of this printing. For more information about the guidelines, contact the American Psychiatric Press Order Department, 1400 K Street NW, Washington, D.C. 20005, 800-368-5777, fax: 202-789-2648.

B. Network Development and Maintenance

For the psychiatric practice accepting capitation for the full range of mental health services, including hospital costs, a network of psychiatrists is required. This is accomplished through contracting with these clinicians to deliver a specified set of services upon referral from the psychiatrist or a designated case manager. A subcontract should specify the rates at which those services will be provided.

Additional capabilities required in the development and maintenance of a clinician network include the following:

B.1. Composition and Geographic Distribution
The psychiatric practice network must be composed of sufficient numbers of psychiatrists who have the following characteristics:

- A diversity of disciplines including psychiatry, psychology, social work, and addictionology;

- A diversity of subspecialties such as child and adolescent treatment, chemical dependency treatment, medication management, family therapy, short-term therapy, grief issues, etc.;

- Sufficient numbers of psychiatrists and other clinicians to ensure that members do not have excessive waiting times for appointments. This is sometimes required in the contract with the MCO, and quick access to outpatient treatment often prevents costly hospitalizations, thus enhancing the financial performance of the capitation arrangement; and

- A sufficient dispersion of psychiatrists and related clinicians in a geographic area to ensure that members do not have inordinately long commutes to treatment. Increasingly, MCOs are requiring that fully capitated psychiatric practices have a certain number of psychiatrists and related clinicians within specified distances of patient locations.

B.2.   Credentialing

In order to protect against liability claims and often as a requirement of the contract with the MCO, the psychiatric practice will be required to credential the clinicians with whom it contracts to ensure they are properly licensed and in good standing in the community. The credentialing function can often be time consuming and expensive, since the psychiatric practice must usually obtain primary source verification of degrees, licenses, and malpractice insurance coverages. Additionally, these files must be maintained and updated at least every two years. Additional requirements may be imposed by the MCO.

B.3.   Training and Communication

A key activity in the maintenance of the network is training each participating psychiatrist in the procedures used by the psychiatric practice in managing the capitated contract. Areas requiring periodic training include the following:

Authorization procedures The participating clinicians must understand how to obtain authorization for services required by patients.

V

Utilization review procedures The psychiatric practice must inform the clinicians and facilities participating in the network about the protocols for conducting ongoing reviews of care delivered to patients. There are usually differing procedures for the review of outpatient and inpatient care. The psychiatric practice may also require use of special protocols for certain procedures, such as psychological testing and ECT, or for certain patients, such as high service utilizers or consistently non-compliant patients. If the psychiatric practice requires the completion of certain forms such as service requests or treatment plans, training must be provided to the network.

Claims filing If the psychiatric practice is paying claims for services delivered by other psychiatrists in its network, the participating psychiatrists must be trained in the proper completion and submission of claim forms. Also, the psychiatric practice's contract with participating psychiatrists should contain language concerning the timely filing of claims.

Quality improvement and outcomes The psychiatric practice may institute an outcomes measurement protocol that requires participation by the participating psychiatrists in its network. Training should be provided to ensure maximum compliance with the protocol. The requirement to participate in such activities should also be specified in the contract.

Monitoring and sanctioning As part of monitoring its participating psychiatrist network, the psychiatric practice may institute specific monitoring protocols such as utilization or cost profiling. Also, the psychiatric practice should develop procedures for sanctioning network psychiatrists who are consistently non-compliant with the management of the contract or who have a significant history of justifiable complaints from patients.

C.   Administrative Processes

In addition to the clinical and network management capabilities, the capitated psychiatric practice may also need other capabilities such as claims payment systems and patient service functions.

C.1.   Claims Processing

Claims payment is required when the psychiatric practice has accepted capitation beyond the scope of its professional services. Usually this requires establishment of a network that enables provision of the services required in its capitated agreements. The psychiatric practice that needs claims payment capability has the following options:

Develop the Capability In-house

Advantages: This method offers the greatest amount of control over the claims payment process. It ensures the highest level of confidentiality along with the quickest access to reports and data necessary for contract management. Alternatives to system purchases include leasing the system from another vendor or from the MCO.

Disadvantages: Setting up this capability can be expensive if the purchase of management information systems (MIS) is required. It also generally requires an additional permanent staffing capability (depending upon the size of the contract and volume of claims) in the form of claims processing staff, clerical support, and information systems support. The psychiatric practice may also have to acquire a state license to operate as a claims processor.

Contract With the MCO

Advantages: This method avoids the initial costs of system implementation and staffing. It also does not require a claims processor license on the part of the psychiatric practice.

Disadvantages: In the long term, it may be more costly to the psychiatric practice, as the MCO will generally charge a portion of the capitation or a transaction fee for the service. Additionally, many psychiatrists feel uncomfortable with the MCO having this level of detail about the costs and utilization associated with the contract. Acquiring reports and data may also be problematic and time consuming.

C.2.   Appeals Process

The capitation agreement may also require the psychiatric practice to have a documented appeals and grievance mechanism to resolve psychiatrist and patient disputes about a number of issues. This capability usually involves three levels:

Level One: The appeal or grievance is received from the MCO and reviewed by the psychiatric practice or its designee. It is wise to have another colleague review the appeal if the psychiatric practice is the subject of the appeal. Notification of the decision is generally given in writing within a certain time frame, usually not to exceed 30 days.

Level Two: If the psychiatric practice or patient disagrees with the findings of the Level One appeal decision, an option is extended for a Level Two appeal. This appeal or grievance is received and reviewed by an independent third party, usually not associated with the psychiatric practice, the participating psychiatrist practice, or the psychiatric practice network. As with Level One appeals, notification of the decision is generally given in writing within a certain time frame, usually not to exceed 30 days.

Level Three: This level is usually the final appeal mechanism available to patients or psychiatrists dissatisfied with the Level One and Two appeal decisions. It is usually conducted by the MCO's appeal and grievance committee, sometimes with an opportunity for hearings and testimony from all parties.

If the psychiatric practice must comply with NCQA guidelines, this appeal procedure must be thoroughly documented and reviewed periodically. Also, the MCO may require certain reports on appeals activity.

C.3.   Quality Improvement

Finally, the capitated psychiatric practice is often required to maintain a formal documented quality improvement (QI) process, including the following:

- Documentation of the plan, its focus, staff responsibilities, and methods for utilizing the information in the improvement of business and clinical processes;

- Targeting and documentation of processes to measure and improve care;

- Development of reliable measures and data collection tools;

- Collection of data on an ongoing basis or for a specific project time period;

- Analysis of the data and the implications for process improvement;

- Development of an action plan to implement the suggested improvements; and

- Continued monitoring of the process over time with feedback to continually revise the plan, measures, and analyses.

To the extent that the MCO retains control of QI, psychiatric practices should be careful to avoid accepting responsibility to participate in procedures that have not been clearly defined or explained in the contract or in any attached manuals or exhibits. Generally, detailed information regarding QI can be found in an MCO's manual or its policies and procedures. The psychiatric practices should carefully review these materials to determine the exact scope of responsibility to be held by each party. Further, they should request the inclusion of language in the contract requiring prior review and notice to the psychiatric practice of any changes in the QI procedures by the MCO.

D.   Management Information Systems

The backbone of any capitated arrangement is the management information system (MIS) supporting the activities. The need for information is perhaps more crucial for a capitated psychiatric practice than for a fee-for-service practice due to the nature of the risk involved. The psychiatric practice that receives capitated premium dollars to manage and deliver the full range of mental health services required by a beneficiary population takes on a level of risk that requires an MIS capable of two-way information transfer between the MCO and the practice. Data such as membership, benefit accumulators, and deductible information must be passed between the psychiatric practice and the insured entity. Internally, the practice system must pass these data to those organizational divisions and staff responsible for managing the benefit.

This model is applicable for practices that manage all benefit functions in-house and for practices that contract with other entities such as third-party administrators (TPAs) for some functions. In either case, the functional systems and data flow must be in place. For assistance with MIS issues and questions, contact the APA's Office of Economic Affairs and Practice Management.

D.1.   General MIS Requirements

The success or failure of a practice in a risk-sharing arrangement such as full capitation is entirely dependent upon the degree to which the practice successfully manages the two key factors of cost per service and utilization of those services by the beneficiary population. This means having access to real-time, accurate information regarding beneficiaries, psychiatrists, and case managers, and having the ability to analyze and communicate key performance data, both internally and externally.

A broad list of possible financial loss points in a fully capitated, risk-sharing environment can illustrate areas where the various practice information subsystems are necessary to avoid losses:

- Authorization or provision of services to ineligible members or to members who have depleted their benefits;

- Inefficient and costly participating psychiatrist networks or service delivery units;

- Overutilization due to inappropriate authorizations, inefficient services, or ineffective case management;

- Inaccurate claims payment, complicated by multiple and complex benefit plans;

- Inability to track claims cost and to project true claims liability (erroneous "Incurred But Not Reported" calculations);

- Faulty capitation pricing arrangements due to lack of data regarding utilization and cost of services; and

- Faulty subcapitation pricing arrangements (with participating psychiatrists) due to the above, complicated by the lack of ability to compare capitation rates with alternative reimbursement rates.

In short, the psychiatric practice MIS should be able to accurately determine who is eligible for benefits, who will deliver the service at what cost, how and when the claims for service will be paid, and how to give accurate utilization and financial information to management and the various customers of the system.

In most cases where the practice is responsible for the full range of services and is using a diverse psychiatrist network, the system should be a mature, comprehensive claims-based system that can be adapted for the particular clinical case management needs of a mental health environment. On the whole, most systems do not have the comprehensive functionality found in true claims systems developed for a managed care environment. In addition to being inherently inefficient, manual systems or home-grown systems become truly ineffective and hazardous when the number of covered lives reaches 20,000 members or above.

At a minimum, the MIS must have capabilities in patient services; clinical case management; network relations and development; claims payment; and financial subsystems, monitoring, and reporting.

Patient services Part of the capitated agreement with the MCO may involve the provision by the psychiatric practice of patient service functions. These functions are defined as those information and support functions provided to both patients and participating psychiatrists or related clinicians regarding benefit eligibility, claim status, clinical questions, complaints, and appeals. The patient service function replaces the one provided by the MCO, particularly if the capitated psychiatric practice is responsible for claims payment for the full scope

V

of services covered by the benefit. In order to be effective, patient services staff must have access to all MISs used in managing and monitoring the activities under the contract. Generally, information is provided to members and participating psychiatrists over the telephone during business hours.

The patient services subsystem must have functionality in group enrollment, benefit design, and patient communications. One critical element is the ability of the MIS to accommodate an increasingly complex mix of benefit plan designs that range from simple benefits with distinct copayments, deductibles, and benefit limits to complex point-of-service (POS) plans with in- and out-of-network options, differing deductibles, and grouped accumulators.

The second critical requirement is the ability of the MIS to accept membership and enrollment information from a variety of sources. Unlike most insured entities, the practice will neither have the infrastructure nor the need to individually enroll members. This requires that the system accept such information electronically, either through network connections or other means of transfer, the most common being magnetic tape loads. The technical process should be able to accept a wide variety of formats and be efficient enough to permit routine membership updates.

Clinical case management The essential MIS requirements to support clinical case management include the ability of the system to allow quick and accurate precertification and concurrent certification by procedure and place of service. This subsystem, often termed an "authorization" or "utilization review" module, must give the psychiatric practice access to relevant benefit plan provisions such as inpatient day limits, outpatient visit limits, annual or lifetime dollar limits, and episode of care limits. Lack of such capability will result in over-authorization of services and subsequent claims liability.

Most older claims systems are not designed for the particular needs of mental health care management; however, there are several options to correct these deficiencies. The first option is to integrate a stand-alone clinical case management system, and the second option is to modify the standard system to include those data elements and functions minimally required for mental health case management.

Network development and relations The two most critical requirements of the network development and relation subsystem are its ability to accommodate a wide variety of contracts with participating clinicians and its ability to capture and report utilization and profiling data on the psychiatrist and clinician network. Regarding the first requirement, the MIS should be able to accommodate contracts involving, at minimum, the following payment arrangements:

- Flat fees;

- Discounts of charged accounts;

- Maximum limits on usual and customary charges;

- Negotiated schedules;

- Diagnosis-related group (DRG) or case pricing, adjusted by age/sex severity;

- Per diems, all-inclusive and global; and

- Capitation.

In situations where the practice chooses to subcapitate to participating psychiatrists for a particular service or geographic area, the system should be able to provide reports comparing the capitation pricing to the reimbursement equivalent of submitted claims. This demand requires that the claims system accept group assignment of capitation arrangements (most claims systems assign capitated psychiatrists on a member-by-member basis as part of the enrollment process, a capability not possessed by most practices). The system should also provide reports such as referral statistics by the psychiatric practice and case manager. It should also facilitate analysis of utilization and comparison across multiple variables, including type of service and diagnosis group, and compare patterns of use on various levels, including peer to peer and individual psychiatrists to total peer group.

Claims payment While the requirements for other subsystems are critical, the functionality of the claims payment subsystem is the point at which everything merges to produce payments for services. In capitated arrangements with large MCOs, the variability of payment rates, psychiatrists, payment mechanisms, levels of care, benefit limits and restrictions, and case management considerations causes the claims payment function to be more complex and demanding than in other environments. To support this critical area, the primary requirement of the claims subsystem is the ability to link with the other subsystems in an automated and real-time fashion. The system should have a variety of automatic edits, security features, and audit trails. It should capture all UB-82 and HCFA 1500 information, calculate deductibles and copays, and place them in correct in/out of plan accumulators. Key automatic linkages should include, at a minimum, service limit calculation and notification, precertification linkage, additional certification linkage, and eligibility checks through membership history links. It should accurately track all benefit limits and provide accumulator information to the authorization and certification subsystems.

In the case where the capitated psychiatric practice is managing an internal claims payment process, it must have monitoring protocols in place that routinely measure key claims-processing activities such as:

- Volume and amount of claims paid;

- Productivity of claims-processing staff;

- Accuracy of processed claims;

- Elapsed time from date of service to claim receipt, from claim receipt to entry into the claims system, from claim receipt to adjudication, from claim receipt to payment, and from claim receipt to check processing;

- Number, status, type, and age of claims that are suspended in the claims system;

- Number, status, type, and age of claims that have been returned to psychiatrists for correction and resubmission;

- Number, type, and value of denied claims;

- Number, type, and value of reversed claims, particularly for services which have been approved upon appeal; and

- Timeliness and efficiency of check processing and mailing.

It should be noted that these indicators should also be required of an external claims payer such as an MCO or a third-party administrator (TPA).

Billing and financials The key requirement for this subsystem is the ability to produce comprehensive financial statements by line of business to evaluate performance on a product-line basis, requiring the capability to support multiple business lines, entities, sites, and locations. In conjunction with this or as an alternative, the system should provide linkages to other general ledger packages and systems already in use by the practice.

These requirements taken together comprise the minimum key requirements for an information system necessary for effective management of risk-sharing contracts, particularly in environments where the practice is fully capitated for all mental health services. What has not been discussed are MIS requirements for integrated practices in which practice management subsystems are integrated with the claims system. Also not discussed were the compelling information system needs to enhance outcome measurement, quality improvement processes and report cards, and other reporting requirements not yet invented. However, the key requirements presented should provide the basis for a system that can accommodate or, at the very least, facilitate these enhancements as they develop.

Following is a list of common reports that should be produced by the information system and used for ongoing management of the capitation:

- **Utilization Summary:** This report provides a management overview of key utilization statistics for the current period.

- **Membership Demographics:** This report provides a summary of employee and dependent counts, showing the age/sex distribution.

- **Outpatient Utilization by Age/Sex:** This report summarizes outpatient visit data by employee, dependent, and age/sex distribution.

- **Inpatient Utilization by Age/Sex:** This report summarizes inpatient admissions by employee, dependent, and age/sex distribution.

- **Distribution of Benefits Paid:** This report shows how benefits were distributed between different types of service, illustrating where the benefit dollar was used under the capitation.

- **Summary of Inpatient Services:** This is a summary report illustrating inpatient utilization for mental health and substance abuse inpatient care, providing data on hospital days per 1,000 lives, admissions per 1,000, and average length of stay.

- **Admissions by Diagnosis and Setting:** This cross-tabulation report shows the distribution of hospital admissions by diagnosis category (mental health vs. substance abuse) and by treatment setting (inpatient, partial hospitalization, and intensive outpatient).

- **Distribution of Utilization:** This report provides data on the most frequently used hospitals and psychiatrists, showing the number of admissions, days/visits, average length of stay, cost per day/visit, total cost, and cost ranking.

- **Summary of Outpatient Services:** This report summarizes outpatient utilization for mental health and substance abuse outpatient visits. Data provided include patients per 1,000 lives, visits per 1,000, and average number of visits per patient treated.

- **Claims Summary:** This report provides a recap of outpatient and inpatient claims received and estimated claims (Incurred But Not Reported [IBNR]), showing total claim dollars, average cost per outpatient visit, and average cost per inpatient day.

- **Patient Recidivism:** This report shows the total number of repeat hospital admissions, also stated as a percentage of initial admissions, for mental health and substance abuse diagnoses.

A wide variety of other reports can be configured as monitoring tools for the capitation. The important point is that the information system used by the practice must be capable of collecting and collating data to facilitate ease and flexibility of reporting.

E.   Financial Monitoring

Perhaps the most critical administrative responsibility of the capitated psychiatric practice is the financial monitoring function, particularly if it is responsible for the entire set of covered services in the benefit plan.

The four main areas of responsibility in prudent financial monitoring are as follows:

E.1.   Capitation Reconciliation

As discussed in Chapter IV, Evaluating and Negotiating a Capitation Contract, the contract should contain provisions for reconciling the capitation payment made to the psychiatric practice. This primarily involves verifying the number of eligible members for each relevant time period and auditing the accuracy of the payments made. This can be done on an ongoing basis if the psychiatric practice is receiving eligibility data electronically and has a database of membership enrollment and disenrollment dates. This activity becomes extremely critical if the psychiatric practice is capitated for a number of different groups with different capitation rates.

E.2.   Claims Payment

Another aspect of capitation reconciliation occurs when the MCO acts on behalf of the capitated psychiatric practice to pay claims to those who are not part of the capitated psychiatric practice but are providing services under its contract. Usually, the amount of claims from participating network psychiatrists paid in a period is deducted from the monthly capitation payment made to the psychiatric practice. In this event, the psychiatric practice must verify the accuracy of these claim payments to ensure proper processing and deductions from the capitation. Careful records of authorizations and covered beneficiaries must be kept to ensure that only services authorized by the psychiatric

V

practice are paid. Also, the psychiatric practice must ensure that the MCO is continually furnished with accurate contract rates for other psychiatrists under contract with the psychiatric practice. If possible, it is preferable that the psychiatric practice develop its own contracts and not rely on the agreements that may be in force with the MCO prior to the capitation.

E.3.   Claims Expense and IBNR Calculation

One of the most crucial aspects of capitated financial reporting is the calculation of fully incurred claims expenses for a period. This is arguably one of the most troublesome aspects of capitation management for psychiatric practices, and it should be reviewed periodically by an actuary with experience in managed mental health plans.

The determination of the true claims expense for a period is a combination of two sets of data:

Amount of claims paid   Value of services delivered
in the period for services   +   in the period for which claims
rendered in the period   have not yet been received.

The latter factor is known as Incurred But Not Reported (IBNR) expenses. Simply stated, IBNR refers to outstanding claims for services that have not been received or have not been captured by the authorization system. An accrual system for these claims is necessary to accurately report claims expenses for a given period.

E.4.   Financial Reporting

For both the psychiatric practice capitated only for professional services and the psychiatric practice capitated for all covered services, the ability to produce accurate and timely financial statements and measures is vital. One of the first important functions is the cost accounting system, which should be able to produce:

- Cost per unit of treatment;

- Cost per course of treatment (episode of care);

- Cost per patient;

- Non-fee-for-service reimbursement; and

- Routine real-time clinical utilization/cost reports including:
  Total Days/Visits per 1,000;
  Days/Visits per 1,000 for Each Level of Care;
  Admissions per 1,000 for Each Level of Care;
  Gross Costs per 1,000 Population for Each Level of Care; and
  Average Length of Stay or Average Visit per Case, in aggregate, by
  diagnosis and presenting problem, by age group, and by level of
  care.

Beyond the traditional financial reports such as income statements,
balance sheets, and cash flow statements,
financial reporting in a managed care
environment should also report other
standard key indicators such as:

Medical loss ratio This is the ratio between costs incurred for health care
services and the premiums received.
A sample calculation is provided at the
right.

Sample Medical Loss Ratio Calculation

- Total Premium Received
  in Month   **$45,000**

- Total Cost for Health
  Care Services   **$26,550**

- Medical Loss Ratio =
  (26,550/45,000) =   **59%**

Per Member per Month Financial Summary

TABLE 18

Item	Current Month	Budget	Variance
Membership	50,000	55,000	(5,000)
Gross Capitation Premium	$4.00	$4.20	($0.20)
Deductions From Premium	$0.00	$0.00	$0.00
Net Capitation Premium	$4.00	$4.20	($0.20)
Cost of Care	$2.35	$2.20	($0.15)
Administrative Costs	$0.55	$0.50	($0.05)
Total Costs	$2.90	$2.70	($0.20)
Profit (Loss)	$1.10	$1.50	($0.40)
Loss Ratio	58.75%	52.38%	(6.36%)

V

Per member per month financial summaries An example is shown in Table 18 (data used are for illustrative purposes only).

A similar presentation of financial results should be completed for year-to-date financial indicators.

Legal and Regulatory Issues for Capitated Psychiatrists

There are legal and regulatory concerns for capitated psychiatrists that differ according to the nature of the capitation arrangement. For example, psychiatrists capitated for the entire mental health benefit and who use a network of clinicians and facilities often face more stringent regulatory concerns than the psychiatric practice that is capitated for its professional services only. It is important to note that these regulatory issues vary significantly from state to state, and the psychiatric practice involved in capitation should work with an attorney specializing in health care and insurance law.

Common to both general types of capitation are insurance and liability issues. A complete set of coverages should be in place to cover the psychiatric practice's activities not only as medical professionals, but also to cover activities in the daily management of care, particularly when the psychiatric practice is reviewing and approving care delivered by other psychiatrists. For more information about legal issues, consider joining the APA's Legal Consultation Plan. Examples of the basic coverages are:

- General liability coverage;

- Professional malpractice coverage;

- Coverage for utilization review activities (this may not be a part of the standard professional malpractice coverage and must be purchased separately); and

- Other standard business coverages.

VI

For the psychiatric practice capitated for its professional services only, the standard regulatory concerns are applicable, such as professional licensing requirements and local and state business permits. Unique to the psychiatric practice capitated for the full range of mental health services are the regulatory issues specific to the acceptance of risk and the payment of claims, such as whether any licensure or general insurance is needed, in addition to third-party administrator (TPA) licensure (for payment of claims) or a utilization review license for case management. Because of the extreme variability from state to state, a psychiatrist considering entering a capitated contract would be well advised to consult an attorney who specializes in health care or insurance law.

Most importantly, the psychiatric practice capitated for all services must often obtain licensure from the state department of insurance to accept risk. It is vital that these requirements be explored with competent counsel, as the definitions of a "risk-bearing entity" vary significantly from state to state. These requirements are in place to protect the covered beneficiaries in the event of a default by the risk-bearing entity, and as such, they often have significant capital reserve requirements. States have generally viewed independent clinicians capitated for direct professional services as being exempt from these regulations. The thinking underlying this exemption was that in the event of significant negative financial results, the psychiatrist would only be required to provide his or her own labor to provide the contracted services. There would be no obligation on the part of the practice to pay claims to others for services.

For those psychiatric practices accepting risk for all services and who use a network of clinicians for the delivery of those services, however, a different set of regulations often apply. In these cases, states are increasingly viewing these arrangements as assumption of "insurance risk," and therefore falling under the insurance licensing requirements. The acquisition of such licenses can be an expensive and time-consuming process. Again, the psychiatric practice should make use of competent legal counsel and should explore alternatives available in the language of the contract with the MCO.

Other regulatory issues involve the applicability of utilization review and third-party administrator licenses. Most states have adopted utilization review legislation requiring any entity performing such activities to acquire a license from the state and provide regular reports to the appropriate state agency. Some states also require psychiatrists who have claims payment responsibilities and functions to acquire a TPA license. In most cases, these licenses are not difficult or expensive to acquire.

Other regulatory issues involve the accreditation of psychiatrists by two organizations: the Utilization Review Accreditation Commission (URAC) and NCQA. Generally, these standards apply only to psychiatrists accepting capitation for the full range of benefit services. At this point in managed mental health, it is not often a requirement that the capitated psychiatrist acquire these licenses and certifications. However, if the MCO with whom the psychiatric practice contracts is currently seeking NCQA certification, the psychiatric practice will often have significant administrative and reporting requirements.

The Dilemma of Quality in Capitated Systems

A. The Conflict of Incentives

In any system of health care financing, there are incentives to design treatment services that maximize financial return for the psychiatric practice. The traditional fee-for-service structure was criticized for its incentive to over-treat and over-charge. The most common criticism of capitation is the incentive to under-treat. Both criticisms are valid, and both systems are subject to abuse.

In arrangements where the psychiatric practice is capitated, there are some distinct advantages and opportunities to manage the financial environment in the best interest of the patient, the plan, and the psychiatric practice. The primary advantage is that the capitated psychiatrist has a degree of freedom to tailor care to the needs of the patient in a way that was difficult if not impossible under the fee-for-service system. The capitated psychiatrist may have the following advantages:

- Psychiatric practices have an opportunity to decrease the utilization review burden, particularly for its own services (in this type of arrangement, the responsibility for utilization review shifts totally to the psychiatric practice).

- Through claims data, the opportunity to "get the whole picture" about an episode of care for a patient.

- Through case management, the opportunity to organize a multi-faceted and, if necessary, multi-disciplinary treatment plan for the most efficient and effective outcome for the patient. Also, through careful and attentive case management, the capitated psychiatrist has the opportunity to enhance the professional collaboration of independent clinicians to a degree rarely possible in a fee-for-service environment.

There are also disadvantages to capitation:

- Conflicts with peers may arise due to the new role as utilization manager.

- There exists the prospect of experiencing significant negative financial consequences due to an overutilization of services, an underestimation of the administrative requirements for effective risk management, or a poorly crafted contract with the payer.

- Financial incentives to limit care may create a conflict of interest.

B.   Satisfaction and Outcomes Measures

One of the mechanisms to assist the psychiatric practice in managing the negative incentives of capitation is a well-developed system of acquiring feedback from patients and other clinicians. Measures of patient and clinician satisfaction can be powerful tools to monitor the quality of service and the process of care management. A suggested protocol for measuring satisfaction is as follows:

- On an ongoing basis, measure the satisfaction of the patient with the authorization and referral process. This can be done by the distribution of a simple survey instrument such as the SF-36 at the point of intake or contact.

- For a sample of patients referred to treatment, measure their satisfaction with the treating clinician. This can be done six weeks after the initial referral and can also serve as a measure of patient follow-through.

- For all hospitalized patients, measure the satisfaction with the attending psychiatrist through discharge interviews or questionnaires.

- At least twice a year, measure the satisfaction of other clinicians with the authorization, referral, and claims payment processes. This can be done in focus groups or through distribution of a questionnaire.

More robust measures of the quality of the capitation arrangement are outcomes programs designed to measure the extent and nature of patient improvement. There are several widely available instruments that are becoming standard tools in the measurement of patient outcomes such as the SCL-90, the BASIS-32, and the Outcome Questionnaire. There are an increasing number of proprietary systems such as the COMPASS system, BEHAVIORisk, and others that are gaining acceptance. The implementation of such systems is rapidly becoming a requirement of purchasers.

Conclusion

Capitation has a long history in the economics of medicine. Only recently has it gained popularity as more and more of the United States' population has moved into managed health care models. Psychiatrists have found themselves competing with other mental health disciplines for patient referrals, and many feel pushed to a limited practice niche of medication management and hospital care. As a result, psychiatrists have begun to explore the opportunities presented by assuming risk for mental health services in both the public and private sectors. Using the resources of the APA's Office of Economic Affairs and Practice Management, Legal Consultation Plan, Consultation Service, and the local District Branches, the psychiatrist treading into these new waters can negotiate these arrangements with confidence and a reasonable degree of success.

The experience and training of today's psychiatrist place him or her in the primary leadership position for these endeavors. Adequately prepared, a psychiatric group practice can effectively compete for risk contracts in today's market, and the results can be very satisfying from a cash flow/profit perspective. But perhaps more importantly, psychiatrists may reclaim autonomy in practice once again.

Appendix 1: Determination of Claim Liability: Medical vs. Psychiatrist Claims

Introduction

The intent of this section is to establish guidelines to help avoid claims-paying disputes in cases where multiple diagnoses are present and/or in which non-psychiatric services and/or psychiatrists are used.

Definitions

Psychiatrist/Psychiatric Professional A licensed or certified psychiatrist, addictionologist, psychologist, psychiatric social worker, or certified alcoholism counselor who has contracted with the psychiatrist to provide mental health services to patients.

Medicine or Physical Refers to physical medicine physicians (i.e., family practitioners, internists, gastroenterologists, etc.) or medical-surgical units established to care for patients with physical illnesses.

Plan The insurance plan, employer, or third party with whom the psychiatrist has contracted to provide mental health management services.

Hospitalization The service (i.e., the plan or psychiatrist) providing the primary treatment for which the patient has been hospitalized will be financially responsible for the hospital room and board charges, i.e., the psychiatrist when the primary treatment is mental and being provided by a psychiatrist; the plan when the primary treatment is physical and being provided by a primary care practitioner (PCP) or a

82

Appendix 1:
Determination of Claim Liability:
Medical vs. Psychiatrist Claims

IX

non-psychiatric/addictions physician. Individual physician charges and charges for tests the physician orders or causes to be ordered will be the responsibility of the service to which the physician belongs, i.e., the psychiatrist when the physician is a psychiatrist; the plan when the physician is a plan PCP or other plan psychiatrist.

The following guidelines will be used in utilization review and in processing claims when the services rendered include a combination of mental health and physical health care:

a. When a patient is admitted with a primary physical diagnosis and a mental health consultation is requested, the psychiatrist will be financially responsible for the consultation.

b. When a patient is admitted for the treatment of a physical problem and there is a concomitant psychiatric problem, the physical care rendered will be the responsibility of the plan. If the patient is medically cleared and transferred to a psychiatric unit, the psychiatrist will assume responsibility at that point. For example, if a patient ingests a toxic substance in a suicide attempt and requires physical care in an ICU, the plan will be responsible for the patient's care until the patient is medically cleared and transferred to a psychiatric unit. If physical care continues when the patient is on a psychiatric unit, the physical health care portion of the claim, including tests ordered by the PCP or non-psychiatric/addictions physician, will be the responsibility of the plan.

c. When a patient is admitted with multiple diagnoses, including both mental and physical diagnoses, the plan and the psychiatrist will be responsible for their respective portions of the claim. For example, if a patient is being treated for alcoholism with a secondary diagnosis of hepatitis, the care rendered for the hepatitis by a PCP or medicine consultant, including ancillary charges, will be the responsibility of the plan; the care rendered by a mental health professional, including ancillary charges, will be the responsibility of the psychiatrist. Financial responsibility for the hospital room and board will be determined by where the patient is housed and who is the primary caregiver, i.e., if the patient is admitted to a psychiatric unit under the care of a

Appendix 1:
Determination of Claim Liability:
Medical vs. Psychiatrist Claims

83

psychiatrist, the psychiatrist will be responsible; if the patient is admitted to a medical-surgical unit under the care of a PCP or other plan psychiatrist, the plan will be responsible.

d. When inpatient detoxification requires treatment on a medical-surgical unit by a non-psychiatrist, it shall be considered a plan expense and will not be the clinical or financial responsibility of the psychiatrist.

e. If a patient is admitted for a physical complaint, but the physical evaluation does not lead to a physical diagnosis and a psychiatric diagnosis is then assigned to the case, the care rendered, other than for psychiatric consultations, will be the responsibility of the plan. When the patient is transferred to a psychiatric unit and the primary caregiver is a psychiatrist, the psychiatrist will be financially responsible. For example, if a patient is admitted for evaluation for pain of unknown etiology, but no organic etiology is identified and the patient is then given a diagnosis of psychogenic pain, the care rendered, other than for psychiatric consultation, will be the responsibility of the plan. If the patient is then transferred to a psychiatric unit, the care will become the responsibility of the psychiatrist.

f. When the above guidelines are insufficient, the following additional general principles will be used to determine claim responsibility:

- What is the primary cause for hospitalization? Which condition could only be treated in a hospital setting?

- What does the cover sheet on the medical record list as a primary diagnosis for this admission?

- Is the attending physician of record a psychiatrist or a PCP/medicine consultant?

- Has the patient been admitted to a psychiatric or a medical/surgical unit?

- Who is the primary caregiver?

- What condition is causing the patient to remain in the hospital and who is treating this problem?

IX

- In the event that a good faith effort by the plan and the psychiatrist does not resolve the question of payment responsibility, the disputed charges will be split 50/50, i.e., 50% to the psychiatrist and 50% to the plan.

Emergency Room If an enrollee is referred or self-refers to an emergency room, the cost of the emergency room evaluation shall be the plan's. If psychiatric consultation is requested, the psychiatrist will pay for the cost of the psychiatric assessment and/or treatment. The costs of all ambulance transfers from the emergency room in these instances shall be the plan's.

Neurological Testing Neurological testing is one of several diagnostic procedures used to determine organic brain disease or deficit or readiness for certain surgical procedures. Neurologists are in the best position to assess whether testing would be useful, such as with a brain scan, EEG, etc. Such testing should only be approved by the PCP or neurologist and paid for by the plan. If such testing is performed as part of a psychiatric evaluation for a psychiatric condition, the psychiatrist will approve and pay the claim.

Biofeedback A psychiatrist may use biofeedback as an adjunctive modality (like one might use hypnosis) in the course of treatment for certain DSM-IV diagnoses, such as anxiety, panic, or phobic disorders, in conjunction with a standard mental health treatment modality. If used as the primary or only treatment modality, biofeedback will not be covered unless so stated in the plan document.

Biofeedback has been demonstrated to be effective in the treatment of conditions that are primarily physical in nature, such as migraine or tension headache, Raynaud's disease, chronic pain, etc. Although the psychiatrist may endorse the use of biofeedback in such treatment, the plan must bear the cost.

Outpatient Treatment As with hospitalization, individual physician charges and charges for tests and/or other ancillary services the physician orders or causes to be ordered will be the responsibility of the service to which the physician belongs, i.e., the psychiatrist when the

Appendix 1:
Determination of Claim Liability:
Medical vs. Psychiatrist Claims

85

physician is a psychiatrist; the plan when the physician is a plan PCP or medicine consultant. Again, the following general principles will be used to determine claim responsibility:

- What is the primary cause for treatment or the services rendered?

- What does the cover sheet on the medical record list as a primary diagnosis for the patient?

- Is the attending physician of record a psychiatrist or a PCP/ medicine consultant?

- Who is the primary caregiver?

Attention-Deficit Disorder The individual physician charges and charges for tests and/or other ancillary services the physician orders or causes to be ordered will be the responsibility of the service to which the physician belongs, i.e., psychiatrist when the physician is a psychiatrist; the plan when the physician is a plan PCP or medicine consultant.

Appendix 2: Instructions for Using the Capitation Worksheet to Estimate a Capitation Rate

American Psychiatric Association
Mental Health Capitation Demonstration Model

Disclaimer: This mental health capitation demonstration model is for educational purposes only. The calculation methodology has been designed and developed to teach psychiatrists about the interrelationships between mental health utilization, mental health service cost, and managed care capitation rates. This demonstration model is not intended to supplant the use of actuarially sound tools and consultation in the calculation of mental health capitation rates.

The corresponding file for the text you are reading is named INSTRUCT.WPD. It is a WordPerfect file and can also be found on the Worksheet diskette. Please review this file before using the Worksheet file. The Worksheet file is named WKSHEET.XLS, and it is a Microsoft Excel file.

Capitation is often called a "population-based" payment method because the psychiatrist or psychiatric group is paid a fixed amount per member for all members in a covered group.

> **For example:**
>
> | | |
> |---|---:|
> | *Number of Covered Members:* | *25,000* |
> | *Capitation Rate Paid to Psychiatric Group, per Member per Month:* | *$3.75* |
> | *Monthly Capitation Payment to Psychiatric Group:* | *$93,750* |

X

Essentially, the capitation payment made to a psychiatric group is a single fee that covers both the net claims cost and administrative costs (which include both overhead and profit). In most capitated mental health payment arrangements, the claims costs include all costs of mental health and chemical dependency treatment at all levels of care—from outpatient services to acute hospitalizations. Administrative costs include both profit and overhead, which are the non-clinical costs of managing the services provided to the group of eligible individuals. Typical overhead costs include rent, utilities, telecommunications, information systems, insurance, and staff members who are not directly involved in providing clinical services.

This Mental Health Capitation Demonstration Model uses a fee-for-service (FFS) methodology for estimating the per-member-per-month (PMPM) capitation rate. The method combines the use of the historical FFS utilization of services by members coupled with an estimate of the current costs to provide those services.

Information You Will Need to Use the Capitation Demonstration Disk

The following steps will guide you through the use of this spreadsheet in the estimation of a capitation rate.

Section 1: Determine the Number of Members in the Plan

In a health maintenance organization or other managed care plan, the number of "members" in the plan is the number of enrolled individuals. (NOTE: In an employer-sponsored health plan or an insurance company health plan, the number of "members" must be calculated. In these plans, the number of members in the plan is the number of employees/insureds multiplied by the dependency ratio—the average number of members in the employee/insureds' families.)

> **For example:**
> *The number of members in a group that has 12,000 employees and an average family size (dependency ratio) of 2.8 would be "33,600" members (12,000 × 2.8).*

Enter the number of members in the group	

Section 2: Estimate the Utilization Rates and Average Length of Stay (ALOS)

For each category listed below, enter the historical experience data provided by the plan and/or your estimate of the impact your clinical management will produce. The first value required is "penetration rate" by level of care. This is an estimate of the number of members the group expects to access the level of care. This estimate should be expressed as a percentage.

For example:
If the historical experience of the group shows that half of a percent of the members use Inpatient Mental Health services in a year, the penetration rate would be ".005."

Psychiatric groups also need to estimate the average length of stay (ALOS), or the average number of visits for outpatient services, by level of care. These values should be entered under ALOS.

Level of Service	Penetration Rate	ALOS
Inpatient Mental Health		
Partial Hospitalization Mental Health		
Alternative Residential Mental Health		
Outpatient Mental Health		
Inpatient Chemical Dependency		
Partial Hospitalization Chemical Dependency		
Alternative Residential Chemical Dependency		
Outpatient Chemical Dependency		

The worksheet will calculate the number of admissions, total days or visits expected, and a set of per 1,000 numbers to be used in the cost portion of the worksheet.

Section 3: Estimate Your Overhead Costs

Every capitation contract will have overhead costs associated with contract management, whether they are dedicated staff, equipment, or

X

other administrative support services. Estimate the costs associated with each contract management function and incorporate them into the capitation rate calculation. Express the values for staff members in terms of Full Time Equivalents (FTEs) per month. A sample list of categories has been provided. You can change these to more accurately reflect the overhead cost breakdowns of your practice or program.

For example:

Two medical records technicians will be required to manage services for a particular group. With salary and benefits, each is paid $24,000 per year. Therefore, the appropriate entries would be "Medical Records Technicians," "2" FTEs, and "2,000."

ESTIMATE YOUR OVERHEAD COST

Sample Categories	Your Categories	Number of FTEs or Units	Cost per FTE or Unit per Month
Director of Clinical Services			
Executive Medical Director			
Case Management Staff			
Secretarial Staff			
Provider Relations Staff			
Finance Staff			
Claims Processing Staff			
Member Services Staff			
MIS Staff			
Marketing Staff			
QI Staff			
Rent and Utilities			
Telephone System			
MIS Acquisition/Upgrade			
Stop-Loss Insurance			
Legal and Consulting			
Licensing/General Ins.			

X

Section 4: Net Claims Cost

"Net claims cost" is the total cost to the psychiatric group for all clinical services delivered to members of the group. To determine these costs, enter the average cost per unit of service (either the actual charge or the anticipated cost) in the spreadsheet, by level of care. If the psychiatric group is purchasing these services from another provider organization, enter the unit cost of the purchased services (for example, the rate with the local hospital is $500 per day). If the psychiatric group is providing these services, enter the fully allocated cost of providing the service (for example, the average cost for the group practice to deliver an outpatient mental health visit is $90 per hour). Such estimates may include the "averaged" costs of a variety of disciplines and clinical specialties. These figures, along with the previous estimates of utilization, are used to calculate gross cost per member per month.

To determine net claims cost per member per month, the psychiatric group must also factor into the cost the effects of payment of deductibles and copayment. *[For illustrative purposes, this model assumes that there is a single fixed-dollar copayment per admission. There is no deductible assumed for outpatient services. The model also assumes that there is a fixed-dollar copayment per unit of service. In reality, there are a host of complicated arrangements for deductibles and copayments— on all levels of care, at fixed dollar amounts, at percentage of cost, based on number of visits, per case and annual. When calculating a capitated rate for a competitive bid, a psychiatric group must factor in the effects of these complicated benefit plan design issues.]* Enter the amount of the deductible per admission for the plan year and the copayment per visit for each level of care. Both the deductible and the copayment should be entered as a dollar amount, not as a percentage.

For example:

For the level of service, Inpatient Mental Health, if the cost per unit is $450.00, the deductible per admission is $50.00 and the copayment per day is $75.00, enter "450," "50," and "75" in the appropriate columns for Inpatient Mental Health.

X

Level of Service	Cost per Unit	Deductible Factor	Copay Factor
Inpatient Mental Health			
Partial Hospitalization Mental Health			
Alternative Residential Mental Health			
Outpatient Mental Health			
Inpatient Chemical Dependency			
Partial Hospitalization Chemical Dependency			
Alternative Residential Chemical Dependency			
Outpatient Chemical Dependency			

Section 5: Final Capitation Pricing

Enter the percent of profit margin to the final capitation pricing formula in Section 5. The profit margin is expressed as a percentage of the net claims cost.

For example:

If the psychiatric group would like a profit margin on the cost of clinical services of 4.0%, enter "4.0" in the profit margin entry column.

Profit Margin	

With the profit margin, the psychiatric group has entered the last data required to get an initial estimate of a capitated mental health rate. The next step for most groups is to test the rate against other known benchmarks. The American Psychiatric Association has a set of capitation rates in the publication *The Capitation Handbook*. For a more in-depth discussion of capitation and pricing mechanisms, please consult this monograph, *The Psychiatrist's Guide to Capitation and Risk-Based Contracting*. In addition, this monograph contains a glossary of terms specific to capitation and risk-based payment arrangements.

APA Resources and Services for Psychiatrists Working in Managed Care

XI

Psychiatrists in need of more information or help with managed care and other professional issues can contact numerous American Psychiatric Association (APA) resources.

APA's Consultation Service—202-682-6203

APA's Legal Consultation Plan—202-682-6064

APA's Managed Care Help Line—800-343-4671

APA's Office of Economic Affairs and Practice Management—
202-682-6212

The APA's address is 1400 K Street, NW, Washington, D.C. 20005.

Capitation and Risk-Based Contracting Bibliography

American Psychiatric Association: *Capitation Handbook.* Washington, DC: American Psychiatric Association, 1995.

Barber, R. & Jones, W., et al. (1996) Capitating physician group practices. *Healthcare Financial Management,* Volume H, p. 46.

Bruder, P. (1996) Capitation: breaking rice bowls. *Hospital Topics,* Volume 74, p. 7.

DeMarco, W.J. & Garvey, T.J. (1986) *Going Prepaid: A Strategic Planning Decision.* Englewood, CO: Center for Research in Ambulatory Health Care Administration.

Goldstein, D. (1996) *Building and Managing Effective Physician Organizations Under Capitation.* Gaithersburg, MD: Aspen Publishers, Inc.

Keene, R.D. & Naus, F.F. (1994) *Negotiating Managed Care Contracts.* New York, NY: McGraw-Hill, Inc.

Kleiman, M. (1996) Preparing for capitated hospital services. *Healthcare Financial Management,* Volume H, p. 40.

Kongstvedt, F.F. (Ed.) (1993) *The Managed Health Care Handbook,* Second Edition. Gaithersburg, MD: Aspen Publishers, Inc.

Melek, S.P. & Pyenson, B.S. (1995) *Actuarially Determined Capitation Rates for Mental Health Benefits.* Washington, DC: American Psychiatric Association.

Neal, P.A. (1986) *Management Information Systems for the Fee-for-Service/ Prepaid Medical Group.* Englewood, CO: Center for Research in Ambulatory Health Care Administration.

XII

Pherson, P. (1996) 8 steps to making capitation work. *Hospitals & Health Networks*, Volume 70, p. 59. Chicago, IL: American Hospital Publishing Inc.

Samuels, D.I. (1996) *Capitation: New Opportunities in Healthcare Delivery.* Chicago, IL: Irwin Professional Publishing.

Schafer, E.L., Olson, C.J. & Gocke, M.E. (1987) *Evaluating the Performance of a Prepaid Medical Group: A Management Audit Manual.* Englewood, CO: Center for Research in Ambulatory Health Care Administration.

Sulger, J. (1996) Establishing reserves for capitation contracts. *Healthcare Financial Management*, Volume H, p. 52.

Sutton, H.L. Jr. & Sorbo, A.J. (1993) *Actuarial Issues in the Fee-for-Service/ Prepaid Medical Group.* Englewood, CO: Center for Research in Ambulatory Health Care Administration.

Wolf, K. & Kreb, R. (1996) Actuary data: What's in it for you? *ASHA*, Volume 38, p. 32. Rockville, MD: American Speech Language & Hearing Association.

Wrightson, C.W. Jr. (1990) *HMO Rate Setting and Financial Strategy.* Ann Arbor, MI: Health Administration Press Perspectives.

Yennie, H. (July/August 1994) Who's minding the data: information system requirements for participating in at-risk contracts. *Behavioral Healthcare Tomorrow,* Volume 3, No. 4, p. 21.

Zinser, G.R. (July/August 1994) Behavioral health at-risk contracting—a rate development and financial reporting guide. *Behavioral Healthcare Tomorrow,* Volume 3, No. 4, p. 27.

Capitation and Risk-Based Contracting Glossary

Actuary A person trained in the insurance field who determines policy rates, reserves, and dividends as well as conducts various other statistical studies.

Adjustable Premium Usually used in connection with guaranteed renewable health policies in which the premium is subject to change based on classes of insured.

Administrative Services Only (ASO) An arrangement under which an insurance carrier or an independent organization will, for a fee, handle the administration of claims, benefits, and other administrative functions for a self-insured group.

Admissions per 1,000 A measure used to evaluate utilization management performance that is calculated by taking the total number of admissions from a specific group (e.g., employer group, or group for which the psychiatrist or payer are at risk) for a specific period of time (usually one year), dividing it by the average number of covered members or lives in that group during the same period, and multiplying the result by 1,000. This is calculated for mental health in aggregate and by modality of treatment (e.g., inpatient, residential, and partial hospitalization).

Adverse Selection Disproportionate enrollment into a plan by individuals with the potential for higher health services utilization than projected for an average population. An older population and impaired or chronically ill individuals are considered adverse risks. Adverse selection may cause premiums to be too low to cover actual plan experience.

Age/Sex Rating A method of structuring capitation payments based on enrollee/membership age and sex.

All-Payer Contract An arrangement allowing for payment of health services delivered by a contracted psychiatrist regardless of product type (e.g., HMO, PPO, indemnity) or revenue source (e.g., premium or self-funded).

Alliances Purchasing pools responsible for negotiating health insurance arrangements for employers and/or employees. Alliances use their leverage to negotiate contracts that ensure that care is delivered in economical and equitable ways. (Also sometimes referred to as health insurance purchasing cooperatives or health plan purchasing cooperatives.)

Allowable Costs Charges for services rendered or supplies furnished by a psychiatrist that qualify as covered expenses.

97

XIII

Alternative Delivery System (ADS) A method of providing health care benefits that departs from traditional indemnity methods. An HMO, for example, can be said to be an alternative delivery system.

Ancillary Charge The fee associated with additional service performed prior to and/or secondary to a significant procedure, such as lab work, X rays, and anesthesia; or a charge in addition to the copayment that the member is required to pay, such as to a pharmacy for a prescription that has been dispensed in nonconformity with the plan's maximum allowable cost list.

Anniversary The beginning of a subscriber group's benefit year. A subscriber group with a year coinciding with the calendar year would be said to have a January 1st anniversary.

Annual Maximum The total combined inpatient and outpatient dollar benefit available to a plan member during the course of his or her plan year, calculated based on the rates paid to plan psychiatrists, exclusive.

Attrition Rate Disenrollment expressed as a percentage of total membership. An HMO with 50,000 members experiencing a two percent monthly attrition rate would need to gain 1,000 members per month in order to retain its 50,000-member level.

Average Daily Census The average number of hospital or health institution inpatients (other than newborn) each day throughout a given period. The census is calculated by dividing the number of patient days during a period by the number of calendar days in the period.

Average Length of Stay (ALOS) Average number of patient days of service rendered to each inpatient (excluding newborns) during a given period. Varies for patients by diagnosis, age, hospital efficiency, etc. One measure of use of health facilities.

Balance Billing A psychiatrist's billing of a covered person for charges above the amount reimbursed by the health plan (i.e., the difference between billed charges and the amount paid). This may or may not be appropriate, depending upon the contractual arrangements between the parties.

Base Capitation A stipulated dollar amount to cover the cost of health care per covered person, less mental health/ substance abuse services, pharmacy, and administrative charges.

Benchmarking An ongoing measurement and analysis process that compares administrative and clinical practices, processes, or methodologies of an organization or an individual with others. The goal is to learn the best practices of others in order to improve. Terms often used are administrative benchmarking and clinical benchmarking.

Beneficiary The person designated or provided for by the policy terms to receive benefits under the insurance contract.

Benefit Year A 12-month period that a group uses to administer its employee fringe benefits program. A majority of subscribers use a January through December benefit year. A benefit year, however, may not match the fiscal year used by a group.

Capitation A stipulated dollar amount established to cover the cost of health care services delivered for a person. The term usually refers to a negotiated per capita rate to be paid periodically, usually monthly, for the delivery of all health services required by the covered person under the condition of the psychiatrist contract.

Carve-Out A separate financing and delivery structure established for a particular group of benefits typically provided by an indemnity or HMO plan. Example: A mental health benefit may be carved out, and a specialized vendor selected to supply these services on a stand-alone basis. These arrangements are usually provided for a fixed fee per subscriber or per member per month. Also sometimes referred to as single service plans (SSP). See Capitation.

Case Mix The relative frequency and intensity of hospital admissions or services reflecting different needs and uses of hospital resources. Case mix can be measured based on patients' diagnoses or the severity of their illness, the utilization of services, and the characteristics of a hospital.

Claims Completion A measure used to evaluate the performance of the claims payment function, usually calculated by subtracting the date of receipt of the claim from the date the claim is adjudicated as paid by the payer. A common industry standard is a 14-day claims turnaround. (Synonyms: elapsed time, turnaround time.)

Claims Lag An analysis, usually performed by an actuary, which allocates the actual dollars paid to the months in which the services are performed. Claims lag analyses are used to determine completion rates for claims payment performance and are integral in the calculation and projection of claims expenses for a given period.

Coinsurance The portion of covered health care costs for which the covered person has a financial responsibility, usually according to a fixed percentage. Coinsurance often applies after first meeting a deductible requirement.

Community Rating A method of determining a premium structure that is not influenced by the expected level of benefit utilization by specific groups, but by expected utilization by the population as a whole. Everyone in a specified community would pay the same premium for the same package of benefits, regardless of age, sex, medical history, lifestyle, or place of residence. An adjusted community rating is a community rating that is influenced by group-specific demographics.

Comorbidity Coexisting (usually chronic) conditions that may affect overall health and functional status beyond the effect(s) of the condition under consideration.

Continuum of Care A range of clinical services provided to an individual or group that may reflect treatment rendered during a single patient hospitalization or may include care for multiple conditions over a lifetime. The continuum provides a basis for analyzing quality, cost, and utilization over the long term.

Contract An agreement executed by a subscriber group. The term may be used in place of subscriber when referring to penetration within a given subscriber group. Also used to designate an enrollee's coverage.

Contract Mix The distribution of enrollees according to contracts classified by dependency categories; for example, the number or percentage of singles, doubles, or families. Contract mix is used to determine average contract size.

Coordination of Benefits (COB) Establishes procedures to be followed in the

XIII

event of duplicate coverage, thus assuming that no more that 100% of the costs of care are reimbursed to the patient.

Copayment A cost-sharing arrangement in which a covered person pays a specific charge for a specified service, such as $10 for an office visit. The covered person is usually responsible for payment at the time the health care is rendered. Typical copayments are fixed or variable flat amounts for physician office visits, prescriptions, or hospital services. Some copayments are referred to as coinsurance, with the distinguishing characteristics that copayments are flat or variable dollar amounts and coinsurance is a defined percentage of the charges for services rendered. Also called copay.

Cost-Effectiveness The degree to which a service or a medical treatment meets a specified goal at an acceptable cost and level of quality.

Cost-Sharing A general set of financing arrangements via deductibles, copays, and/or coinsurance in which a person covered by the health plan must pay some of the costs to receive care. See Copayment and Coinsurance.

Cost-Shifting The practice by some psychiatrists of redistribution of the difference between normal charges and amounts received from certain payers by increasing charges made to other payers.

Covered Expenses Hospital, medical, and miscellaneous health care expenses incurred by the insured that entitle him/her to a payment of benefits under a health insurance policy. Found most often in connection with major medical plans, the term defines, by either description, reasonableness, or necessity, the type and amount of expense that will be considered in the calculation of benefits.

Credentialing A process of review to approve a psychiatrist who applies to participate in a health plan. Specific criteria and prerequisites are applied in determining initial and ongoing participation in the health plan.

Critical Pathways Charts showing the key events that typically lead to the successful treatment of patients in a certain homogeneous population. They organize, sequence, and time the major interventions of nursing staff, physicians, and other departments for a particular case type (such as asthma), subset, or condition.

Current Procedural Terminology (CPT) A list of medical services performed by psychiatrists and other physicians. Each service and/or procedure is identified by its own unique 5-digit code. CPT has become one of the industry's standards for reporting of physician procedures and services.

Days (or Visits) per 1,000 A measure used to evaluate utilization management performance that is calculated by taking the total number of days (for inpatient, residential, or partial hospitalization) or visits (for outpatient treatment) received by a specific group for a specific period of time (usually one year), dividing it by the average number of covered members or lives in that group during the same period, and multiplying the result by 1,000.

Deductible Annual expenses a subscriber has to pay before an insurance plan covers health care costs. These often apply to a subscriber and his or her family in total.

Dependent Any member of a subscriber's family who meets the applicable eligibility requirements of the health plan and who has enrolled in the plan in accordance with its enrollment requirements.

Diagnosis-Related Groups (DRGs) A system used by Medicare for classification of inpatient hospital services based on principal diagnosis, secondary diagnosis, surgical procedures, age, sex, and presence of complications. This system of classification is used as a financing mechanism to reimburse hospitals and selected other psychiatrists for services rendered.

Direct Contracting Individual employers or business coalitions contract directly with psychiatrists for health care services with no HMO/PPO intermediary. This enables the employer to include in the plan the specific services preferred by their employees.

Discounted Fee-for-Service An agreed-upon rate for service between the psychiatrist and payer that is usually less than the psychiatrist's full fee. This may be a fixed amount per service, or a percentage discount.

Employee Assistance Program (EAP) Services designed to assist employees, their family members, and employers in finding solutions for workplace and personal problems. Services may include assistance for family/marital concerns, legal or financial problems, elder care, child care, substance abuse, emotional/stress issues, violence in the workplace, sexual harassment, dealing with troubled employees, transition in the workplace, and other events that increase the rate of absenteeism or employee turnover, lower productivity, and raise other issues that impact an employer's financial success or employee relations management. EAPs can also provide voluntary or mandatory access to mental health benefits through an integrated mental health program.

Employee Retirement Income Security Act of 1974, Public Law 93-406 (ERISA) This law mandates reporting and disclosure requirements for group life and health plans.

Encounter Face-to-face meetings between a covered patient and a psychiatrist where services are provided or rendered. The number of encounters per member per year is calculated as the total number of encounters per year/total number of members per year.

Enrollment The total number of covered persons in a health plan. The term also refers to the process by which a health plan signs up groups and individuals for membership, or the number of enrollees who sign up in any one group.

Exclusive Provider Organization (EPO) A managed care organization that designates a single provider where services may be rendered. The term is derived from the phrase preferred provider organization (PPO). However, whereas a PPO generally extends coverage for non-preferred provider services as well as preferred provider services, an EPO provides coverage only for contracted providers. Technically, many HMOs can also be described as EPOs.

Experience Rating The process of setting rates based partially or in whole on previous claims experience and projected required revenues for a future policy year for a specific group or pool of groups.

Explanation of Benefits (EOB) A description, sent to patients by health plans, of benefits received and services for which the health care psychiatrist has requested payment.

Family Deductible A deductible that is satisfied by the combined expenses of all covered family members. For example,

XIII

a program with a $25 deductible may limit its application to a maximum of three deductibles ($75) for the family, regardless of the number of family members. See Deductible.

Fee-for-Service A traditional means of billing by a health professional for each service performed, referring to payment in specific amounts for specific services rendered (as opposed to a retainer, salary, or other contract arrangements). In relation to the patient, it refers to payment in specific amounts for specific services rendered.

Fee Maximum The maximum amount a participating psychiatrist may be paid for a specific health care service provided to plan members under a specific contract. A comprehensive listing of fee maximums used to reimburse physicians and/or other psychiatrists on a fee-for-service basis is called a fee schedule.

Fee Schedule A listing of fees or allowances for specific medical procedures, which usually represents the maximum amounts the program will pay for specific procedures. (Synonym: Table of Allowances.)

First-Dollar Coverage Feature of a health care plan in which the plan does not require its participants to pay any deductibles or copayments before benefits are received.

Flat Fee per Case Flat fee paid for a patient's treatment based on their diagnosis and/or presenting problem. For this fee, the psychiatrist covers all of the services the patient requires for a specific period of time.

Flat Schedule A type of benefits schedule in group insurance under which everyone is insured for the same benefits, regardless of salary, position, or other circumstances.

Functionality A quality of life indicator that relates to whether a patient has the potential to respond to treatment options and, as a result, be able to function in a normal life.

Guidelines Systematically developed statements on medical practice that assist practitioners and patients in making decisions about appropriate health care for specific medical conditions. Guidelines are frequently used to evaluate appropriateness and medical necessity of care. Terms used synonymously include practice parameters, standard treatment protocols, and clinical practice guidelines. Outcomes can be used as information to modify or improve guidelines.

HCFA Health Care Financing Administration. The federal agency responsible for the administration of Medicaid and Medicare programs.

Health Maintenance Organization (HMO) An organization that provides comprehensive medical care for a fixed annual fee. Physicians and other health professionals often are on salary or on contract with the HMO to provide services. Patients are assigned a primary care doctor or nurse as a gatekeeper, who decides what health services are needed and when. There are four basic models of HMOs: group model, individual practice association, network model, and staff model.

Health Plan A network of hospitals, doctors, clinics, and others that provides a comprehensive range of health services.

Health Plan Employer Data and Information Set (HEDIS) A core set of performance measures to assist employers and other health purchasers in understanding the value of health care purchases and evaluating health plan performance.

Used by the National Committee for Quality Assurance to accredit HMOs.

Health Status An overall evaluation of an individual's degree of wellness or illness, with a number of indicators, including quality of life and functionality. A form often used for this purpose is SF-36.

Hospital Affiliation A contractual relationship between a health plan and one or more hospitals whereby the hospital provides the inpatient benefits offered by the health plan.

IBNR Incurred But Not Reported. Refers to the contingent liability of a plan for the cost of services that have been received by patients but for which no claim for payment has been received. IBNR projections form the basis for the reserves needed by plans to cover expenses as they are calculated by the benefit provisions.

Indemnity An insurance program in which the insured person is reimbursed for covered expenses. It is a traditional health insurance plan with little or no benefit management, a fee-for-service reimbursement model, and few, if any, restrictions on psychiatrist selections.

Individual Practice Association (IPA) A health care model that contracts with an entity, which in turn contracts with physicians, to provide health care services in return for a negotiated fee. Physicians continue in their existing individual or group practices and are compensated on a per capita, fee schedule, or fee-for-service basis.

Integrated Delivery System A generic term referring to a combination of practitioners who deliver health care in an integrated way. Some models of integration include physician hospital organization, a management service organization, group practice without walls, integrated

psychiatrist organization, and medical foundation.

Joint Commission on Accreditation of Healthcare Organizations (JCAHO) A private, not-for-profit organization that evaluates and accredits hospitals and other health care organizations providing home care, mental health care, ambulatory care, and long-term care services.

Legal Reserve The minimum reserve a company must keep to meet future claims and obligations as they are calculated under the state insurance code. The reserve amount is usually determined by an actuary.

Length of Stay (LOS) The number of days that a covered person stays in an inpatient facility.

Lifetime Maximum The total combined inpatient and outpatient dollar benefit available to a plan member during the course of his or her lifetime, calculated based on the rates paid to plan psychiatrists, exclusive.

Management Service Organization (MSO) A legal entity that provides practice management, administrative, and support services to individual physicians or group practices. An MSO may be a direct subsidiary of a hospital or may be owned by investors.

Maximum Benefits The maximum annual or lifetime benefits to which a plan member is entitled.

Maximum Limits Maximum amount payable under a health plan for each cause, for each year, or for lifetime.

Medicaid A program, adopted in 1965, of health insurance for eligible disabled and low-income persons, administered by the federal government and participating states. The program's costs are shared by the federal and state governments, and paid for by general tax revenue.

Medicare A nationwide, federally administered health insurance program that covers the costs of hospitalization, medical care, and some related services for eligible persons. Medicare has two parts: Part A covers inpatient costs and is also called Supplementary Medical Insurance Program. Part B covers outpatient and all physician costs for Medicare patients.

Medicare Supplement Policy A policy guaranteeing that a health plan will pay a policyholder's coinsurance, deductible, and copayments and may provide additional health plan or non-Medicare coverage for services up to a predefined benefit limit. In essence, the policy pays for the portion of the cost of services not covered by Medicare. Also called Medigap or Medicare wrap.

Morbidity An actuarial determination of the incidence and severity of sicknesses and accidents in a well-defined class or classes of persons.

Network Model HMO An HMO type in which the HMO contracts with more than one physician group, and may contract with single- and multi-specialty groups. The physician works out of his/her own office. The physician may share in utilization savings but does not necessarily provide care exclusively for HMO members.

Organized Delivery Systems Proposed networks for psychiatrists and payers that would provide care and compete with other systems for enrollees in their region. Systems could include hospitals, primary care physicians, specialty care physicians, and other psychiatrists and sites that could offer a full range of preventive and treatment services. Also referred to as accountable health plans (AHP), coordinated care networks (CCN), community care networks (CCN), integrated health systems (IHS), and integrated service networks (ISN).

Outcomes Measures Assessments which gauge the effect or results of treatment for a particular disease or condition. Outcomes measures include the patient's perception of restoration of functional status, as well as measures of mortality, morbidity, cost, quality of life, patient satisfaction, and others.

Outcomes Management A term coined by Paul Ellwood in a seminal article in 1988. Definitions vary, but it generally involves collection and analysis of results of medical processes and performances according to agreed-upon specifications and the use of that information to optimize health care provisions through the collaborative efforts of patients, payers, and psychiatrists.

Outlier A patient who varies significantly from other patients in the same DRG, such as by having a longer or shorter length of stay, dying, leaving against medical advice, etc.

Out-of-Area Benefits Those benefits that the plan supplies to its subscribers when outside the geographical limits of an HMO. These benefits usually include emergency care benefits plus low indemnity payments for non-emergency benefits. Most plans stipulate that area services for emergency care will be provided until the subscriber can be returned to the plan for medical management of the case.

Paid Claims The dollar value of all claims paid, i.e., hospital, medical, surgical, etc., during the plan year, regardless of the date that the services were performed.

Participating Provider A provider who has contracted with the health plan to provide medical services to covered persons. The provider may be a hospital, pharmacy, other facility, or a physician who has contractually accepted the terms and conditions set forth by the health plan.

Pathways Multi-disciplinary treatment intervention roadmaps for a specific diagnostic group which promote effective use of resources, decreased length of stay, and collaboration.

Patient Days Accumulated total, for the reporting period, of the number of patients in a hospital each day (excluding newborns). A patient day is one patient in one hospital bed for one day.

Payer Any individual or organization that pays for health care services—including insurance companies and various government programs such as Medicare and Medicaid.

Percentage of Occupancy The ratio of actual patient days to the maximum possible patient days as designated by bed capacity, during any given period.

Per Diem An agreed-upon rate per inpatient, residential, or partial hospitalization day that is all-inclusive. All ancillary services, in addition to therapies and room and board are included in this rate. Sometimes the psychiatrist services are included, and in these situations the per diem is referred to as global. It is not usually the case, however.

Physician-Hospital Organization (PHO) A legal entity formed and owned by one or more hospital and physician groups in order to obtain payer contracts and to further mutual interests. Physicians maintain ownership of their practices while agreeing to accept managed care patients under the terms of the PHO agreement.

The PHO serves as a negotiating, contracting, and marketing unit.

Point-of-Service (POS) A provision that allows patients in managed care plans that limit choice of doctors and hospitals to seek treatment outside of the plans. Patients who use this option typically are required to pay more.

Preferred Provider Organization (PPO) A variation of the traditional fee-for-service care arrangement representing a group of physicians, dentists, and/or hospitals and other practitioners that contracts with employers, unions, or third-party administrators to provide employees with services at competitive rates. Employees have free choice among the physicians in a PPO arrangement. The employee is not penalized or prevented from using his or her regular physician, even if that physician does not participate in the PPO. PPOs usually provide incentives for participation, such as a competitive rate structure. In addition, PPOs generally use primary care physicians to assure that hospitalization occurs only when absolutely necessary, with extensive concurrent utilization review.

Primary Care Network (PCN) A group of primary care physicians who have joined together to share the risk of providing care to their patients who are covered by a given health plan.

Primary Care Physician (PCP) A physician, the majority of whose practice is devoted to internal medicine, family/general practice, and pediatrics.

Primary Data Information obtained from medical records or other primary sources of clinical findings, such as diagnostic tests and physical examination results.

Professional Review Organization (PRO) A physician-sponsored organiza-

XIII

tion charged with reviewing the services provided to patients. The purpose of the review is to determine if the services rendered are medically necessary; provided in accordance with professional criteria, norms, and standards; and provided in the appropriate settings.

Prospective Reimbursement Any method of paying hospitals or other health care psychiatrists for a defined period (usually one year) according to amounts or rates of payment established in advance.

Quality The features of a product or service that bear on its ability to satisfy the stated or implied needs of the user, or consumer. Quality assessment should include consumers' evaluations of how well a product or service meets their needs and expectations with respect to process, outcomes, and perceived value.

Reinsurance A type of protection purchased from insurance companies specializing in underwriting specific risks for a stipulated premium. Typical reinsurance risk coverages are 1) individual stop-loss; 2) aggregate stop-loss; 3) out-of-area; and 4) insolvency protection.

Retrospective Review Determination of medical necessity and/or appropriate billing practice for services already rendered.

Risk The chance or possibility of loss. In insurance terms, it is the probability of loss associated with a given population. The term may also include physicians, who may be held at risk if hospitalization rates exceed agreed-upon thresholds. The sharing of risk is often employed as a utilization control mechanism within the HMO setting.

Risk Analysis The process of evaluating expected medical care costs for a prospec-

tive group and determining what product, benefit level, and price to offer in order to bear the amount of acceptable risk.

Risk Factors Conditions that influence a person's health and are capable of provoking ill health, including inherited or biological, environmental, and behavioral risk factors.

Risk-Sharing A method by which premiums and costs of medical protection are shared by plan sponsors, participants, and psychiatrists.

Self-Insurance An entity itself assumes the risk of coverage and makes appropriate financial arrangements rather than purchasing insurance from a third party and paying a premium for this coverage.

Standard Benefit Package A specified set of minimum medical benefits available to all persons.

Stop-Loss Insurance Insurance coverage taken out by a health plan or self-funded employer to provide protection from losses resulting from claims greater than a specific dollar amount per covered person per year.

Third-Party Administrator (TPA) An independent person or corporate entity (third party) that administers group benefits, claims, and administration for a self-insured company/group. A TPA does not underwrite the risk.

Third-Party Payers The insurer who pays for the services provided to a patient.

Triple Option Multiple option plans which typically include indemnity, PPO, and HMO plans through one insurer. Triple option plans, in theory, prevent "adverse selection" by placing all employees in a single-risk pool.

Unbundling Separately packaged units that might otherwise be packaged together. For claims processing, this includes psychiatrists billing separately for health care services that might be combined according to industry standards or commonly accepted coding practices.

Underwriter The term generally used applies either to (a) a company that receives the premiums and accepts responsibility for the fulfillment of the policy contract; (b) the company employee who decides whether or not the company should assume a particular risk; or (c) the agent who sells the policy.

Underwriting The process by which an insurer determines whether or not and on what basis an application for insurance will be accepted.

Usual, Customary, and Reasonable (UCR) Fees The Usual Fee is that fee usually charged for a given service by an individual psychiatrist to his or her private patient, that is, the psychiatrist's own usual fee. A fee is Customary if it is in the range of usual fees charged by psychiatrists of similar training and experience in an area. A fee is Reasonable if it meets the two previous criteria or, in the opinion of the responsible medical or dental association's review committee, is justifia-

ble considering the special circumstances of the particular case in question.

Utilization The extent to which the members of a covered group use a program or obtain a particular service or category of procedures, over a given period of time. Usually expressed as the number of services used per year per 1,000 persons eligible for the service.

Utilization Criteria The guidelines used to establish the medical necessity and appropriateness of a course of treatment.

Utilization Management The close management of patient utilization of health care services inside a managed health care program.

Utilization Review (UR) A formal assessment of the medical necessity, efficiency, and/or appropriateness of health care services and treatment plans on a prospective, concurrent, or retrospective basis.

Withhold A percentage of payment to the psychiatrist held back until the cost of referral or hospital services has been determined. Physicians exceeding the amount determined as appropriate lose the amount held back.